STROKE REHABILITATION:
THE RECOVERY OF MOTOR CONTROL

Stroke Rehabilitation: The Recovery of Motor Control

Pamela W. Duncan, M.A., P.T.

Assistant Professor
Graduate Program in Physical Therapy
Duke University
Durham, North Carolina

Mary Beth Badke, M.S., P.T.

Associate Director
Research and Education
Physical Therapy Program
University of Wisconsin Hospitals and Clinics
Madison, Wisconsin

YEAR BOOK MEDICAL PUBLISHERS, INC.

CHICAGO • LONDON • BOCA RATON

1 2 3 4 5 6 7 8 9 0 KC 91, 90, 89, 88, 87

Library of Congress Cataloging-in-Publication Data

Stroke rehabilitation.

   Includes bibliographies and index.
   1. Cerebrovascular disease—Patients—Rehabilitation.
2. Motor learning.   I. Duncan, Pamela W.   II. Badke,
Mary Beth.   [DNLM: 1. Cerebrovascular Disorders—
rehabilitation.   WL 355 S921373]
RC388.5.S8565   1987   616.8'106   86-32620
ISBN 0-8151-2936-X

Sponsoring Editor: Stephany S. Scott
Manager, Copyediting Services: Frances M. Perveiler
Production Project Manager: Robert Allen Reedtz
Proofroom Supervisor: Shirley E. Taylor

To the memory of my mother, Trannie E. Woods, who provided me with the right beginning, and in honor of my husband, W. Larry Duncan, who has always supported my efforts.

PAMELA W. DUNCAN

With intense affection and appreciation, I dedicate this book to the memory of my father, Paul Badke, and to the Heavenly Father, who gave me my parents, for it is they who taught me perseverance and faithfully supported me in all my endeavors.

MARY BETH BADKE

Contributors

PAUL BACH-Y-RITA, M.D.

Professor and Chairman, Department of Rehabilitation Medicine, University of Wisconsin Medical School, Madison, Wisconsin

RICHARD BALLIET, Ph.D.

Assistant Professor and Director, Neuromuscular Disabilities Clinic, University of Wisconsin Medical School, Madison, Wisconsin

MARY BETH BADKE, M.S., P.T.

Associate Director, Research and Education, Physical Therapy Program, University of Wisconsin Hospitals and Clinics, Madison, Wisconsin

ELEANOR F. BRANCH, Ph.D., P.T.

Associate Professor, Graduate Program in Physical Therapy, Duke University, Durham, North Carolina

PAMELA W. DUNCAN, M.A., P.T.

Assistant Professor, Graduate Program in Physical Therapy, Duke University, Durham, North Carolina

ROSS L. LEVINE, M.D.

Assistant Professor of Neurology, University of Wisconsin Medical School, Madison, Wisconsin

JACQUELINE MONTGOMERY, M.A., P.T.

Physical Therapy Supervisor, Rancho Los Amigos Hospital, Downey, California

CAROLEE J. WINSTEIN, M.S., P.T.

Department of Kinesiology, University of California, Los Angeles, Los Angeles, California

Preface

For many years, the assessment and treatment of sensorimotor deficits following stroke have been based on clinical observations and empirical evidence. More recently, research in the basic and clinical sciences has given us the opportunity to more scientifically describe the motor deficits and recovery of function following stroke, as well as to critically examine the conceptual and neurophysiologic bases for our treatment approaches. The purpose of this book is to present the "art and science" of stroke rehabilitation by merging new theories with clinical practice. Medical evaluation and management of stroke patients is presented. Current research has been reviewed in order to describe the pathologic and neurophysiologic basis of movement disorders following stroke. Recent theoretical concepts of motor control and learning are discussed and applied to their clinical use in neuromuscular rehabilitation. Determinants of abnormal motor control and strategies for the rehabilitation of motor deficits are described in detail. Valid and reliable methods of motor assessment are also presented. Finally, a thorough approach to the pathokinesiology and management of locomotor deficits is presented.

This book reflects the efforts of many individuals who are experts in stroke research and rehabilitation. The multidisciplinary analysis of the sensorimotor deficits and recovery of function following stroke makes this book a useful teaching tool and reference for practicing physicians, therapists, and other health professionals.

PAMELA W. DUNCAN, M.A., P.T.

MARY BETH BADKE, M.S., P.T.

Acknowledgments

"Tough times never last but tough people do," with a little help from God and their friends. The friends who supported us during this endeavor include Susan Attermeier, who helped keep our thinking straight, Eleanor F. Branch, whose editorial reviews were invaluable, John Hughes, who willingly let us photograph his recovery, Linda Behney, who typed and re-typed the manuscript, and last but not least, all of our patients, who inspired this book.

PAMELA W. DUNCAN, M.A., P.T.

MARY BETH BADKE, M.S., P.T.

Contents

1

Diagnostic, Medical, and Surgical Aspects of Stroke Management*

Ross L. Levine, M.D.

Stroke constitutes the most common disabling and lethal neurological disease of adult life, and one of the most devastating manifestations of atherosclerosis and hypertension. The Cerebrovascular Survey Report of the National Institutes of Neurological and Communicative Disorders and Stroke estimates 400,000–500,000 new strokes occur annually. The estimated financial cost exceeds $7 billion per year, and the human cost is immeasurable.[58]

While coronary artery disease is a frequent occurrence in persons who appear well, stroke develops on a background of cerebral atherosclerosis, established arterial hypertension (70%), coronary artery disease (30%), peripheral vascular disease (30%), diabetes mellitus (15%), and overt congestive heart failure (15%).[62] Because progressive atherosclerotic vascular occlusive disease has obvious manifestations (i.e., atherothrombotic brain infarction, coronary artery disease) and consequences (i.e., disability, death), we have been particularly concerned with multifactorial intervention in our stroke

*This work was supported in part by Veterans Administration merit review grant 821-103.

1

patients. For example, episodes of transient ischemic attacks (TIAs) as warning signs of impending stroke surpass even angina pectoris as premonitory signs of myocardial infarction (MI) or sudden cardiac death.[12]

In this chapter, we keep in mind the multisystem nature of diffuse and progressive atherosclerotic vascular occlusive disease, but will focus primarily on stroke. The hypothetical clinical scenarios are intended to illustrate the principles of stroke management and neurologic care.

EPIDEMIOLOGY

PREVALENCE

Cerebrovascular disease is a major contributor to disability, accounting for at least half the patients hospitalized for neurologic disease. The American Heart Association estimates that there are between 1.5–2.2 million stroke victims each year, a prevalence roughly half that of coronary artery disease.

The great vulnerability of the brain to ischemic damage makes it likely that prevention of stroke, not improved medical and surgical management, is the key to reduction of morbidity and mortality from stroke.[29, 62] The case fatality rate in the acute stroke stages is only 15%, but, of the survivors, at least 50% suffer permanent neurologic disability. A preventative approach to cerebrovascular disease would thus seem necessary, because there has been only limited success of reversing established brain damage.[29]

INCIDENCE

Stroke occurs at a frequency around 0.5–1% per year in the general population over the age of 60 years. Stroke fatalities are exceeded only by heart disease and cancer. While slightly more than 400,000 new strokes occur annually, the incidence of stroke increases steadily with age. For reasons that are not clear, stroke is the only major clinical atherosclerotic manifestation that fails to exhibit a preference for males.

Data from the Harvard Cooperative Stroke Registry[37] and the Framingham Study[61] are in close agreement as to the frequency of stroke subtypes. Between 53–58% of strokes are thrombotic, with 18% of these a result of carotid artery atherothrombosis, 16% from disease of the vertebral-basilar system, and 19% lacunar infarctions involving deep penetrating arterioles. Cerebral embolism accounts for somewhere between 19–31% of all strokes, while hemorrhagic strokes are seen 16–21% of the time.

RISK PROFILE

RISK FACTORS

Progress toward stroke prevention can be recognized, but there is need for many more careful clinical and laboratory studies before the devastation of completed stroke is eliminated.[4] The appearance of stroke or TIA should be defined as failure of prevention. The most significant impact on stroke to date would be risk factor management.[4,62] For example, the potential for prevention has already been demonstrated by the lowered incidence of stroke in hypertensive subjects following detailed antihypertensive therapy. Modification of certain risk factors (i.e., cigarette smoking) also has been demonstrated to improve the prognosis of patients with coronary artery disease. Acceleration in the decline in the incidence and mortality from cerebrovascular disease in recent years is a clear indication that stroke is not an inevitable consequence of aging or genetic constitution.[11,62]

All other therapeutic interventions, then, have to be compared to the diminution of stroke morbidity and mortality and, to a lesser extent, decline in cardiovascular mortality that has occurred since the 1940s. Contributing to these downward in-

TABLE 1-1.

Stroke Risk Factors

ATHEROGENIC	NONATHEROGENIC
Arterial hypertension*	Age and gender
Systolic Hypertension*	Race
Coronary artery disease*	Familial Tendencies
Transient ischemic attacks*	Polycythemia*
Carotid bruits	Alcohol consumption*
Diabetes mellitus	Physical inactivity*
Hyperlipidemia*	Obesity*
Cigarette smoking*	Oral contraceptive use*
Prior stroke	

*Treatment related to decreased stroke incidence has been previously established.

cidence trends are issues of risk factor management (Table 1–1), advances in medical therapy, and improvements in surgical techniques.

SIGNS OF CEREBROVASCULAR COMPROMISE

The two major clinical manifestations that suggest some compromise of the cerebral circulation are asymptomatic carotid bruits (ASBs) and TIAs. There certainly is a growing enthusiasm for early detection and early intervention in both of these conditions. As part of an overall risk factor assessment, we advocate careful historical examination for TIAs as well as auscultation for carotid bruits.

Asymptomatic carotid bruits occur in about 5% of the general population over age 50 years and in as many as 20% of patients who are about to undergo vascular reconstructive procedures such as coronary artery bypass.[24, 64] While it remains controversial as to whether an ASB conveys a significantly increased risk of stroke, it is clear that an ASB is a sign of advanced atherothrombotic disease.

It is estimated that surgically accessible carotid artery atherothrombotic disease of the extracranial circulation accounts for less than 15% of strokes. This is in keeping with the conservative, nonsurgical approach advocated for most patients with ASBs. Once a patient develops a well-defined TIA, however, the risk of subsequent stroke rises to almost 7% per year.[22] In addition, up to 40% of patients with TIAs develop stroke, the majority within 1 year of TIA onsent.

TRANSIENT ISCHEMIC ATTACKS

Case History 1.—A 62-year-old patient presents for further evaluation of recurrent episodes of transient weakness of the right face and arm. These episodes last 10–15 minutes each. Vascular risk factors include hypertension and smoking. Neurologic examination is normal except for bilateral carotid bruits.

DIAGNOSIS, DEFINITION, DIFFERENTIAL

A TIA is a focal reduction in nutrient cerebral blood flow resulting in a short period of neurologic dysfunction from which the individual recovers rapidly without permanent deficit. By definition there is complete recovery of neurologic function within 24 hours, although the majority of TIAs last from 5–20 minutes. As the nature of this phenomenon has been studied, no single underlying mechanism satisfactorily explains the expression in the clinical picture of TIAs.[4]

The patient in case 1 is experiencing carotid ischemic attacks. There is strong clinical and angiographic evidence that links TIAs with all grades of stenosis of the carotid artery [20, 50] and even with atheromatous ulceration of the artery without narrowing.[20] Either flow-limiting or thromboembolic phenomena may be operating given the appropriate conditions. In addition, to understand a TIA one must be able to explain why the fall in blood flow is brief and localized and why, in the affected region, neuronal metabolism can be severely disrupted by ischemia, but can make a rapid and complete recovery.[50]

We are particularly interested in extracranial carotid stenosis, because it is *the* clinical entity most amenable to examination and possible surgical reconstruction. Although quite variable, the symptomatology of carotid TIA in an individual patient tends to conform to a single type. Characteristically repetitive, stereotyped events, TIAs tend to start abruptly, go in flurries, and sometimes disappear without treatment.[29]

The most common variety of carotid TIA affects the middle cerebral artery, as in case 1, or the ophthalmic artery. Any one or combination of the following symptoms is considered a clinical manifestation of carotid TIA: (1) motor (22–70%) or sensory (21–57%) symptoms limited to one limb, one side of the body, or one side of the face; (2) aphasia or dysphasia (16–25%); and (3) retinal ischemia or amaurosis fugax (5–40%).[13, 16, 18, 60] Weakness, clumsiness, or heaviness that involve the face, arm, and leg are the most common motor symptoms of TIA; next in frequency is involvement of the arm alone, face-arm, and arm-leg, in that order.[13]

The presence of unilateral symptoms (i.e., monocular blindness, monoparesis) should be easy to distinguish from the bilateral or alternating symptoms in patients with vertebral-basilar insufficiency (VBI). Combinations of the following symptoms are considered clinical manifestations of VBI: (1) bilateral or alternating motor and/or sensory dysfunction; (2) bilateral visual disturbances, diplopia; (3) dysequilibrium, ataxia, imbalance, or unsteadiness; and (4) dysphagia, dysarthria, or vertigo. Symptoms that are not indicative of TIA include (1) syncope or altered consciousness; (2) dizziness, "wooziness," or giddiness; (3) amnesia alone, confusion alone, vertigo alone, diplopia alone, dysphagia alone, or dysarthria alone; (4) tonic-clonic motor activity; (5) jacksonian march of motor or sensory symptoms; and (6) incontinence.

Risk of stroke appears to be greater in carotid than vertebral-basilar territories,[60] prompting the clinician to make every effort in pinpointing the vascular territory involved in the TIA. Conditions such as focal epilepsy, focal dysfunction in migraine, hypoglycemic reactions, hypertensive encephalopathy, cardiac syncope, and labyrinthine disorders must be included in careful differential diagnostic evaluations of patients presenting with TIA-like phenomena. In addition, reports of patients with transient tumor attacks[49] and transient subdural hematoma[39] attacks complicate the diagnostic process.

NEURODIAGNOSTIC STUDIES

After exclusion of patients with arteritis or hematologic disorders and those with a cardiac source for embolism, the remainder (constituting over 90% of those with transient ischemia) are presumed to have atherosclerotic cerebrovascular disease.[51] In ideal circumstances, all patients with episodes of transient cerebral symptomatology should have a computerized tomographic (CT) head scan. It is thus possible to be sure that a brief reversible focal disturbance is not due to a minor hemorrhage or to a cerebral tumor (Fig 1–1).[29, 39, 51] Up to 25% of patients with TIA will have abnormal results on head CT scan, either indicative of a prior stroke, a mass lesion such as cerebral tumor or abscess, an area of hemorrhage, or a completed stroke with transient signs. The CT scan in case 1 was normal.

Electroencephalography (EEG) may indicate an epileptogenic focus and thereby warrant consideration of a diagnosis of focal epilepsy. If a destructive focus with focal slowing of the EEG background is seen, then localizable cortical damage may be present. The EEG results are almost always normal after a TIA, as in case 1.

Series of patients with TIA studied with magnetic resonance imaging (MRI) should be forthcoming in the neurologic literature. Positron emission tomographic (PET) studies provide a means not only of studying regional cerebral blood flow (rCBF) in patients with TIA, but of determining the physiologic consequences of any alterations in cerebral perfusion by providing information about cerebral perfusion reserve,[31, 32] cerebral blood volume, and localized metabolism.[44]

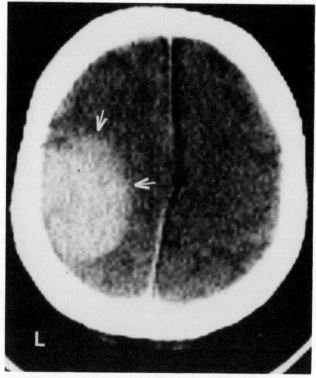

FIG 1–1.
Plain CT scan of a 71-year-old patient who presented with a transient epi-
sode of speech loss and right-sided weakness. A large enhancing menin-
gioma is seen over the convexities of the left cerebral cortex *(arrows).*

Progressive atherosclerotic development of preocclusive
and occlusive lesions in the major cerebral arteries may significantly alter the perfusion to the peripheral arterial beds supplied by each respective stenotic artery. Because the cerebral
vasculature is provided with several potential collateral pathways, the adequacy of these collateral pathways will help determine eventual clinical outcome. With our present PET
techniques,[32] a dynamic sequence of scans initiated during
inhalation constitute the input data necessary for rCBF determination based solely upon measuring fluorine-18-fluorome-

thane ($^{18}FCH_3$) activity in end-tidal expired breaths. Room air (RA) and hypercapnic (CO_2) determination of cerebral perfusion reserve seems to be able to identify those TIA patients with impaired capacity of collateral circulation (Fig 1–2). Further investigations with PET are needed to define different types of TIA according to physiologic criteria and to determine if physiologic measurements are of prognostic value when used in combination with clinical, angiographic, and CT scan findings.[44]

Carotid Doppler/ultrasound studies provide (1) physiologic flow measurements of the extracranial carotid arteries; (2) a flow measurement match to angiographic results; and (3) measurement of the contralateral carotid artery such that an asymptomatic reference point is established, which then can be followed noninvasively.[1] If our patients are deemed unfit for surgical treatment, we do not subject them to angiography; alternatively, all good surgical candidates have definitive invasive studies.[1] We also utilize serial Doppler/ultrasound studies to follow disease regression or progression in all of our vascular patients.

TIAs: MANAGEMENT DECISIONS

GENERAL MEASURES

Identification and control of risk factors such as hypertension and diabetes mellitus are strongly advised. In fact, a diligent program of risk factor modification, especially if the patient agrees to modify his behavior, may be the only plausible therapeutic measure for some patients.

MEDICAL MANAGEMENT

Clinical ischemic vascular disease has a high degree of association with atherosclerosis, and it seems logical to assume that the primary cause of ischemia is decreased blood flow

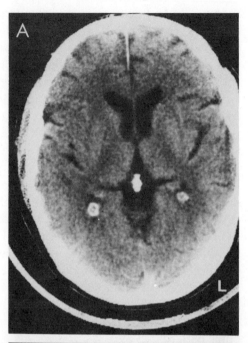

FIG 1–2.
Neuroimages on a 67-year-old patient (series computer code H.N.) who presented with both transient episodes of right monocular blindness and episodes of left body weakness. A plain CT **(A)** is normal. While room air fluoromethane PET images **(B)** appear normal, PET images following hypercapnia **(C)** (see next page) delineate a clear decrease in rCBF in the right hemisphere *(arrows). (Continued)*

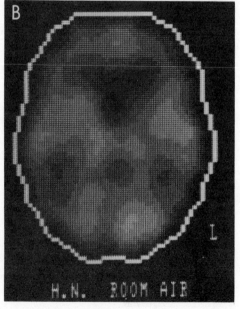

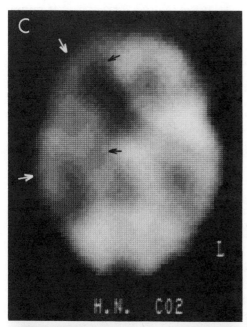

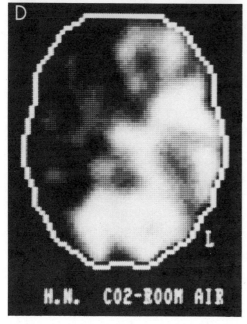

FIG 1–2 (cont.).
The "perfusion reserve" map of CO_2 minus RA data **(D)** also delineates this area at risk of permanent damage.

distal to an atherosclerotic stenosis of an artery.[13, 50, 51] It might
be assumed that the usual event in stroke and heart attack
is an artery-to-artery embolus lodging distal to collaterals or
that platelet-fibrin aggregates or thrombi that are not constant
form over the surface of an atherosclerotic plaque and produce dynamic changes.[19, 50] It is also likely that the atherosclerotic lesions act as triggers for thromboembolic phenomenon. Following this reasoning and similar reasoning that
atherosclerosis entails a progressive, dynamic process of recurrent thromboembolic phenomena, clinicians have assumed
that these ischemic events might be lessened or prevented
by the use of either anticoagulant or platelet-antiaggregate
therapy.[10]

We tend to prescribe antiplatelet therapy for an indefinite
period of time in patients with all forms of ischemic cardiovascular and cerebrovascular disease and in all patients under-
going vascular reconstructive procedures. In addition, data
from various studies using antiplatelet therapy in TIA suggest
that strokes in treated patients are less severe than those in
untreated patients.[21] The choice of antiplatelet vs. anticoagulant treatment, however, remains an empirical matter for indi-
vidual-physician preference. Because a detailed discussion of
specific agents and specific doses is not possible in this chapter, we refer the reader to a number of excellent, readily available reviews on this subject.[10, 14, 15, 18, 42, 53, 59]

Medical management is favored in those patients who have
vertebral-basilar insufficiency; have symptoms in a part of the
brain not supplied by a stenotic artery; or who have a higher
operative risk for reasons of age, intercurrent illness, cardiac
ischemia, hypertension, or diabetes.[51] Surgical management is
favored in those patients who have a localized accessible lesion of the symptomatic internal carotid artery, do not have
severe cardiac ischemia, and will be operated upon by a skilled
vascular surgeon.

SURGICAL MANAGEMENT

Carotid reconstructive surgery via endarterectomy technique remains the procedure of choice for removal of symptomatic stenotic or ulcerated lesions of the extracranial carotid artery.[47] The clearest indication for surgical management of patients with TIA or minor stroke is reconstruction of unilateral carotid ulceration[20] or stenosis with symptoms referable to the artery in question.

Angiography plus carotid surgery should have a combined morbidity plus mortality of 3% or less; otherwise, the patients fare better with medical management alone.[4] Problems in evaluating the efficacy of carotid surgery in ischemic cerebrovascular patients[47, 65] include the following: (1) patients chosen for surgical intervention usually have a better prognosis than those chosen for medical management *(unselected studies);* (2) the efficacy of antiplatelet and anticoagulant agents in relation to each other and to surgical treatment remains largely unknown *(uncontrolled studies);* (3) either flow-limiting or thromboembolic phenomena, or both, may explain the mechanism of cerebral ischemia distal to extracranial stenosis,[19] and it is unknown whether the same therapy applies to both conditions; (4) only up to 40% of patients with TIA develop stroke *(unselected, uncontrolled studies);* and (5) atherothrombotic disease of the surgically accessible carotid artery accounts for only 10–15% of all strokes.

Nonetheless, for patients who have defined carotid disease, with normal or near-normal neurologic status and good surgical risk profiles, and who are willing, we do recommend carotid reconstructive surgery.

MANAGEMENT OF ASYMPTOMATIC BRUITS

The goal of management is to give the patient safe options for reduction of stroke risk while not forgetting that the greatest risk is not for stroke but for myocardial infarction and cardiac death.[2] Reduction of risk factors should be foremost in each clinician's mind during selection of therapy.

We use serial Doppler/ultrasound studies to follow disease progression in patients with asymptomatic bruits. There is a subpopulation of asymptomatic patients who show rapidly progressing atherosclerotic lesions approaching 80% stenosis on serial noninvasive testing. These patients are likely to benefit from prophylactic carotid surgery.[48] Our present approach in ASB patients includes (1) risk factor management; (2) antiplatelet agents; (3) patient education about TIA identification and reporting; and (4) serial Doppler studies. In general, then, the more "inappropriate" the carotid lesion is to the nature of the patient's presentation, the less efficacious is carotid surgery as prophylaxis and the more dubious the benefit-risk ratio.

ACUTE BRAIN INFARCTION

Case History 2.—A 76-year-old patient with hypertension, diabetes, and organic heart disease suffers the abrupt onset of aphasia, right-sided facial and arm weakness, and right hemisensory deficit. His neurologic signs remain dense and unchanged when evaluated 36 hours after onset.

DIAGNOSIS, DEFINITION, DIFFERENTIAL

The diagnosis of acute brain infarction depends upon careful interpretation of clinical history and physical examination, first localizing the brain lesion and then characterizing its type and cause. The patient in case 2 has suffered a completed stroke in the distribution of the left internal carotid artery.

The clinical picture usually will decide the cerebral location. Weakness predominating in the face-plus-arm or leg-only suggests involvement of the carotid artery and cerebral cortex, whereas equal involvement of face-arm-leg suggests a subcortical or brain stem lesion. Sensory impairment is similarly distinguishable. Capsular or subcortical syndromes tend to conform to pure motor or pure sensory syndromes. Inattention or awareness that a stroke has occurred suggests nondominant cerebral hemisphere involvement, whereas dysphasia suggests a dominant hemispheric lesion. Vertigo, ataxia, diplopia, dysarthria, or dysphagia suggest involvement of the vertebral-basilar arteries and the brain stem, although dysarthria and dysphagia can occur in cortical lesions. Disturbances in hemifield vision are difficult to localize in and of themselves. A discussion of each specific arterial syndrome, however, is not possible in this chapter.

Interruption of cerebral blood flow is the most common cause of focal neurologic dysfunction, and the syndromes of acute brain infarction that result provide each clinician with exercises in neural and vascular anatomy.[35] The size of a lesion and the syndrome that it produces depend upon multiple factors that include (1) the individual size of the involved vessel's territory; (2) the duration of the localized circulatory compromise; and (3) the degree of collateral circulation. These factors will be expanded below.

Acute brain infarctions are commonly distinguishable by their ischemic or hemorrhagic nature. The differential diagnosis of a stroke syndrome would then be as follows (1) ischemic (thrombotic, embolic); (2) lacunar; (3) hemorrhagic (spontaneous, aneurysmal, angiomatous); (4) traumatic injury (cerebral contusion, epidural or subdural hematoma); (5) cerebral abscess; and (6) cerebral tumor. A specific diagnosis would thus render a specific management plan; that is, diagnoses such as brain trauma or cerebral neoplasia would warrant completely different therapies.

The following factors help substantiate a bedside diagnosis of ischemic stroke (1) a preceding history of TIAs; (2) underlying atherosclerotic vascular disease; (3) abrupt onset of symptomatology; (4) no history of head trauma; and (5) no evidence of epileptic seizures. The distinction between thrombosis and embolism is so difficult clinically that usually we consider most ischemic strokes as thromboembolic in nature. Once an ischemic stroke is suspected, issues of acute medical stabilization and urgencies of accurate diagnoses arise simultaneously. For the sake of specificity, we will assume that the patient in case 2 is suffering from an ischemic infarct based on thromboembolism and atherosclerosis. The acute stabilization issues are, however, readily applicable to a wide variety of acute brain injury states.

ACUTE MEDICAL STABILIZATION

Our overall goal is to resuscitate areas of brain injury in an attempt to limit the extent of irreversible brain damage. Normalization of all metabolic and physiologic measurements is paramount; focal neurologic dysfunction is usually much more severe with concomitant metabolic derangement such as hyponatremia or uremia. Seizure thresholds are also lowered with the combination of acute brain injuries and metabolic abnormalities.

Systemic blood pressure management is controversial. Initial target mean arterial blood pressures (MABP) of 120 mm Hg are recommended[54] in order to ensure adequate blood flow to ischemically compromised tissue. For patients with long-standing, severe hypertension, the target MABP should be around 130–140 mm Hg, whereas in a young, previously normotensive individual the target MABP might reasonably be even lower than 120 mm Hg.[54] Liberalization of blood pressure to assure tissue perfusion is offset in hemorrhagic stroke where MABPs are lowered aggressively to limit extension of the hemorrhagic process.

Uncontrolled hyperglycemia can induce further tissue destruction by promoting lactic acidosis.[43] The presence of hyperglycemia in acute stroke is also associated with higher mortality, larger infarctions, and more severe clinical disability.[6] Data such as this would thus prompt aggressive normalization of all metabolic measurements.

General medical issues worth accounting for but of unproved significance include (1) keeping the patient with an acute brain injury from eating so as to avoid aspiration pneumonitis until swallowing function can be properly tested with videofluoroscopy[46]; (2) careful cardiac monitoring for myocardial ischemia/infarction, cardiac failure, dysrhythmias, and sources of emboli; and (3) administration of two thirds of the normal amount of maintenance fluids so as to limit potential cerebral edema. Careful clinical studies outlining MABP measurements, glucose levels, fluid volumes, and the like, should be forthcoming in the near future. Once steps toward medical stabilization are initiated, further specific neurodiagnostic examination can be entertained.

NEURODIAGNOSTIC STUDIES

We advocate urgent evaluation in our stroke patients in an effort to make pinpoint, accurate diagnoses whenever possible. The investigation of these patients has been revolutionized by the advent of CT scanning. Scans obtained acutely will be able to distinguish between ischemic and hemorrhagic stroke and to detect nonvascular causes of acute neurologic dysfunction mimicking stroke. Early diagnoses are made to exclude otherwise treatable conditions such as brain abscesses or neoplasms and to study the evolution of tissue changes in infarction and the presence of cerebral edema.

Infarction may be detectable as an area of decreased density on CT in as many as 60–75% of cases. Normal scans are frequently encountered when the lesions are small, such as in lacunar or brain stem infarctions. Acute CT scans in ischemic infarcts are usually negative or may show early edematous changes. The diagnostic yield of CT scanning in ischemic infarcts is at its highest 7 days after the ictus. Areas of decreased density are ill-defined at first, but become more clearly demarcated as time passes (Fig 1–3).

In some 5% of cases, the infarct is isodense or unclearly hypodense and only shows up after contrast enhancement (Fig 1–4). Contrast enhancement in the first week after an ischemic infarct is due to diapedesis of cells from necrotic capillaries;

the more frequently observed late enhancement might be the result of a blood-brain barrier (BBB) disturbance, which in turn is attributed to increased pinocytotic activity of regenerating endothelial cells.[28] Early and persistent enhancement may favor cerebral neoplasia or cerebral infection. Contrast scanning, however, is usually reserved for more atypical presentations where the yield of a tumor diagnosis, for example, would be higher.

Cerebral edema may be seen as soon as day 1 or 2 (see Fig 1–3), but is maximal between days 4 and 7 following ischemic injury and tends to resolve by days 10–20 poststroke. There may be a mass effect with some shift of the midline or obliteration of ipsilateral cortical sulci. Mass effect after 25 days would favor tumor as the cause of the neurologic defect. As already implied, distinguishing stroke from tumor will carry necessary therapeutic implications. Concomitant MRI scanning may also provide valuable information regarding early stroke detection and should be able to distinguish infarction from neoplasm.

Let us assume that the plain CT scan in case 2 was normal on day 2 of stroke. As mentioned, the initial CT scan should be normal and therein should exclude other possibly treatable conditions for the neurologic deficit. An EEG obtained while the CT scan still shows negative results will reveal a slow-wave focus immediately if the overlying cerebral cortex is damaged. Examination of the cerebrospinal fluid (CSF) is rarely performed in stroke anymore. The CSF should be studied in patients with either unexplained fever or with signs of meningeal irritation in order to exclude meningitis or cerebral/subarachnoid hemorrhage. The diagnosis in patients with initially negative results on CT scan is greatly enhanced using early MRI or PET.

Because infarction is evident within 2–6 hours following the ictus, MRI is particularly promising in stroke diagnosis.[55] The spatial resolution of gray and white matter is superior to that of CT, and sodium-MRI images are used to distinguish tumor edema from infarct edema. Tumor edema tends to outline the white matter of the hemisphere at a distance from the mass lesion and has a finger-like pattern; infarct edema has a more uniform, localized appearance. Also, MRI identifies a multiplicity of vascular infarctions in many patients in whom plain CT scan identifies a single lesion, if any. Whether the presence of multiple infarcts without dementia influences the clincial picture or prognosis remains to be clarified in a careful prospective study.

Serial CT scans may be necessary to localize the area of infarction and may help predict prognosis and determine the utility of vascular therapy. Early MRI scanning may have a surprisingly high yield in lesion localization (Fig 1–5) and may someday supplant conventional CT scan as the procedure of choice in stroke diagnosis. Positron scanning is also emerging as an exciting way of imaging regional blood flow and localized cerebral metabolism. Early PET scanning also has a high yield in lesion localization (Fig 1–6). In addition, PET may provide a method to determine if cerebral ischemia in an individual stroke is reversible or irreversible.[31] Further studies correlating clinical and radiographic data with quantitative regional measurements of cerebral physiology are needed in order to determine if either acute interventional therapies in stroke add to the reversibility of cerebral ischemia or improve clinical outcome.

ISCHEMIC INFARCTION-MANAGEMENT DECISIONS

THERAPY FOR ISCHEMIC INFARCTIONS

We are faced with countless potential therapies for stroke victims, many of which have no proved clinical efficacy. In many situations there is no predictable therapy entertained other than medical stabilization. This is particularly true in major strokes where patients have severe deficit, although they may benefit from active, prompt rehabilitation. Patients with

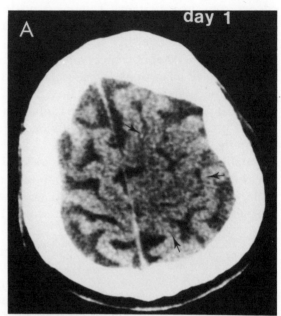

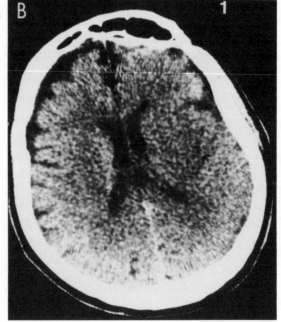

FIG 1–3.
Serial plain CT images on a
64-year-old patient with an
acute left infarction. Scans
on *day 1* postinfarction **(A,
B)** show early loss of sulcus
patterns **(A,** *arrows*)
because of edema.
(Continued.)

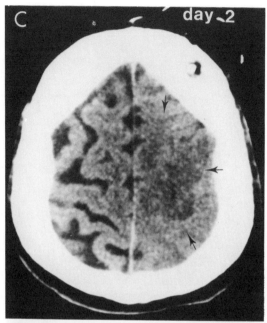

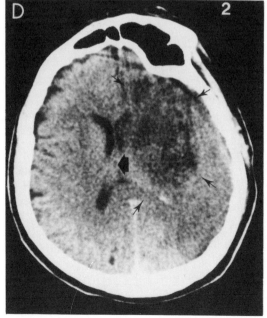

FIG 1–3 (cont.).
Scans on *day 2* **(C, D)** are
much clearer in delineating
the area of infarction (**D,**
arrows) and the severe mass
effect (**D,** *large arrow*).

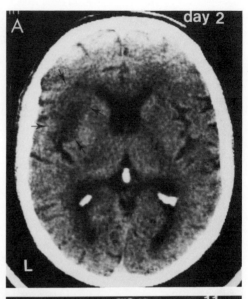

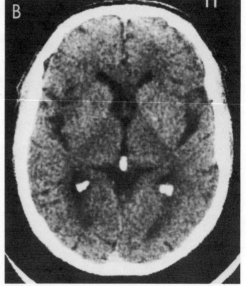

FIG 1–4.
Plain CT image on the 2nd day postinfarction **(A)** showing an area of hypodensity *(arrows)* in this 76-year-old patient. The hypodensity has resolved somewhat by *day 11* **(B)**, but enhances following contrast administration **(C,** *large arrow) (see next page). (Continued.)*

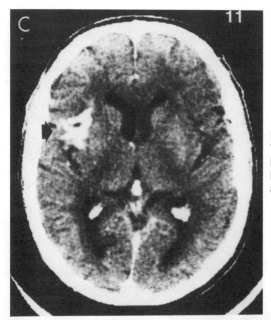

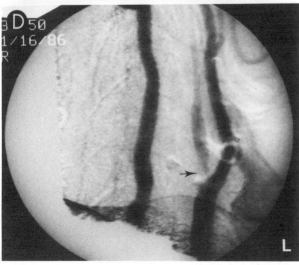

FIG 1–4 (cont.).
This patient was found to have a critical stenosis of the left internal carotid by angiography (**D,** *arrow*).

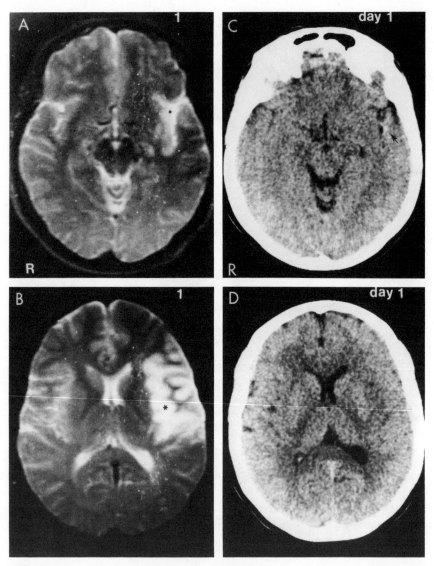

FIG 1–5.
Concomitant plain CT and MRI images following an embolic occlusion of left middle cerebral artery branches. Day *1* MRI images **(A, B)** clearly show the infarct *(asterisk)*. Corresponding level day 1 CT images **(C, D)** show only a widening of the sylvian fissure **(C,** *arrow). (Continued.)*

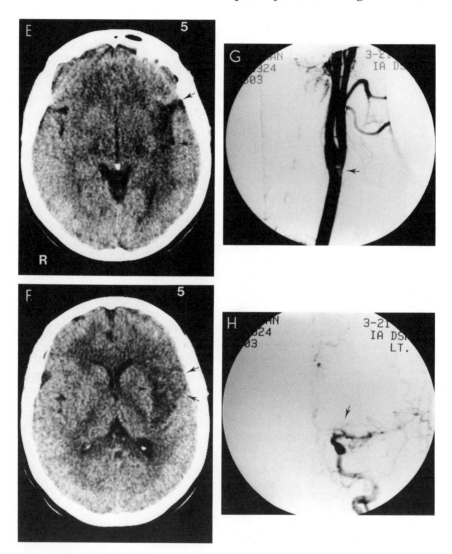

FIG 1–5 (cont.).
Day 5 CT images **(E, F)** reveal a similar area of hypodensity *(arrows)*. Left carotid angiography **(G)** shows a complex ulcer *(arrow)* as the presumed embolic source and intracranial images **(H)** show the occlusion of middle cerebral artery branches *(arrow)*.

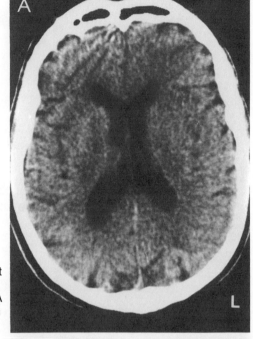

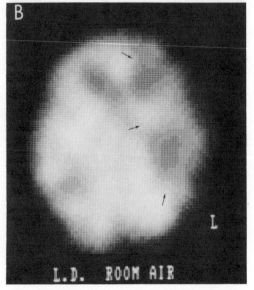

FIG 1–6.
Neuroimages on a 71-year-old patient (series computer code L.D.) studied 30 days postinfarct in the left cortex. Plain CT at days 1 and 30 **(A)** is normal. RA fluoromethane PET suggests an rCBF decrease **(B,** *arrows),* especially in the interhemisphere differences image **(C,** *downward arrow)* (see next page). *(Continued.)*

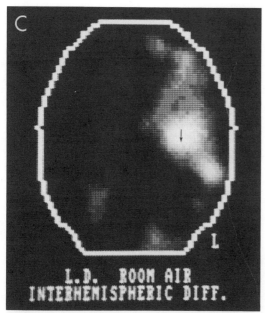

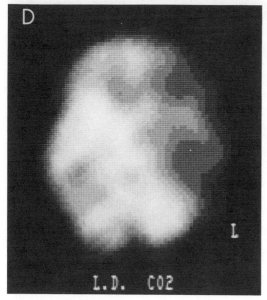

FIG 1–6 (cont.).
Hypercapnic PET shows a
generalized increase in rCBF
because of vasodilation
except in the injured area (**D,
E,** with *downward arrow*)
(see next page). *(Continued.)*

FIG 1–6 (cont.).
"Perfusion reserve" as defined by CO_2 minus RA is decreased (**F**, *downward arrow*). An area of paradoxical decrease or "steal" is also seen **(F)** and is due to failure to vasodilate an already maximally vasodilated ischemic region.

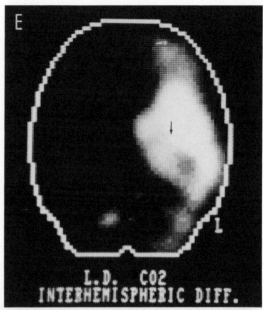

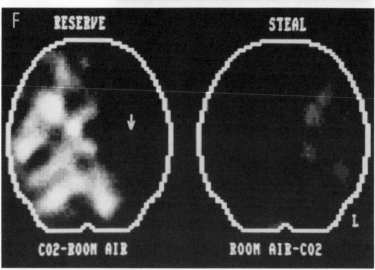

TIA and minor stroke are at a high risk for developing major strokes and usually benefit from aggressive investigation and management; up to one third of such patients deteriorate neurologically, prompting the term "stroke-in-progression." Deteriorating stroke calls for prompt investigation and specific action directed toward the most likely cerebral or systemic factor before the deficits become severe and irreversible. Young patients with stroke have better powers of recovery.[25]

Evidence from clinical observation, neurophysiologic changes, neurochemical studies, and neurohistology indicates a wide spectrum of potentially reversible events preceding brain cell death.[25] However, no specific drug treatment for cerebral infarction is of proved value, and surgical management following stroke is equally dubious.

The therapeutic options available in ischemic infarction are outlined in Table 1–2. We tend to entertain such therapies in research protocols only. A few principles, however, do deserve emphasis.

Osmotic therapy is beneficial in head injuries and following hemorrhagic stroke. It is especially useful in treating severe vasogenic edema. Corticosteroids are surprisingly used worldwide, but have never been proved effective. In addition to being costly, side effects such as gastrointestinal bleeding and hyperglycemia can clearly worsen stroke morbidity.

When we entertain antithrombotic therapy with heparin/ warfarin sodium we are particularly careful in defining exactly what we are treating. Cerebral angiography is frequently necessary in a subset of stroke patients to either demonstrate an embolic branch-artery occlusion or suggest thrombosis-in-progression. The absence of major atherosclerotic changes on cerebral angiography combined with clinical evidence of cardiac dysfunction (i.e., atrial fibrillation, myocardial wall akinesis) may lead to the conclusion of cardiac source and consequent anticoagulation.

Stroke or thrombosis-in-progression is really a mosaic of conditions with a pathologic span large enough to include lacunar infarcts, distal field infarctions, thrombotic and embolic

TABLE 1–2.

Treatment of Ischemic Infarction

TYPE	PURPOSE	RESULTS
Osmotherapy Urea, mannitol	Reduce blood volume, reduce ICP,* improve rCBF†	Short-lived therapeutic effect; especially useful with preherniation
Steroids	Reduce vasogenic edema	Dangerous and ineffective, overused
Antithrombotic		
Heparin	Prevent progressive thrombosis, propagation of clots	Controversial, beneficial only if progressive thrombosis proved, overused.
Warfarin sodium	Prevent second cerebral embolism in cardiac-embolic source patients	Effective, somewhat risky if not watched carefully
Antiplatelet	Decrease secondary platelet thrombi, preventive	Downward trend of second stroke occurrence.
Thrombolytic	Reverse thrombosis	Dangerous, feared because of hemorrhagic potential, needs study
Autoregulatory		
Vasodilation	Improve deficient perfusion	Not effective, may actually worsen because of "intracerebral steal"
Vasoconstriction	Shunt blood into areas of regional ischemia	Not effective
Hemorrheologic		
Dextran 40	Decrease viscosity, improve microcirculation	Early results encouraging if given less than 24 hours postinfarction
Experimental		
Barbiturates	Decrease cerebral metabolism and ICP	Not effective unless given before infarction
Fluorocarbons	Increase oxygen-carrying capacity and reduce viscosity	Encouraging, nonrandom trials
Naloxone	Improve microcirculatory flow	Encouraging, nonrandom trials
Prostacyclin	Decrease platelet aggregation, vasodilator	Encouraging, nonrandom trials

*Intracranial pressure.
†Regional cerebral blood flow.

infarcts, and cerebral hemorrhages.[17] Heparin therapy should thus be restricted even in this subclassification of stroke patients. Cerebral and systemic disorders contributing to stroke-in-progression include (1) a progressing thrombus interfering with anastomotic circulation and extending the area of ischemia; (2) continuing accretions to a thrombotic nidus slowly obliterating the vessel lumen; (3) spread of cerebral edema; (4) recurrent emboli; and (5) concurrent metabolic, acid-base, water-electrolyte disorders, and concurrent infectious processes.[17]

It is also important to recognize that most stroke victims worsen before they improve. Hemorrheologic therapy with agents such as dextran 40 is meant to improve cerebral microcirculation and demonstrates promise in early reports.[63] It is especially useful if initiated within 24 hours following the ictus in a period before vasogenic edematous worsening of the insult has maximized. Many of the other experimental therapies are geared at prompt reversal of ischemia in the early stages of stroke evolution.[25] Again, once vasogenic edema and BBB permeability have maximized, it is unlikely that stroke therapy will be very effective.

The genesis of ischemic cerebral edema is multifactorial, and the relative importance of these many factors may vary throughout the stages of infarction.[40] Cerebral edema is defined as a relative increase in brain water content and brain tissue volume. In ischemic lesions the initial event is intracellular or cytotoxic edema and affects either white or gray matter (or both). It is characterized by the accumulation of intracellular fluid without leakage of proteins or extravasation of BBB proteins. Cytoxic edema develops over the initial 24 hours poststroke and is then complicated by extracellular or vasogenic edema. There has been no stroke therapy that has successfully treated cytoxic edema once it has formed. The cerebral blood vessels undergo characteristic changes that permit leakage of proteins into the extracellular spaces, particularly in the white matter.[30] Vasogenic edema begins to develop between the 24 and 48 hours poststroke, is maximal around the 4th to 7th day, and starts to resolve thereafter. Thus, while vasogenic edema may lessen with diuretic agents or steroids, neither therapy will influence the initial impact of the cellular damage.

In the patient with cerebral infarction, clinical examination alone cannot distinguish between areas of severe ischemia with energy failure, high extracellular potassium concentrations, and developing infarction, and areas with less severe ischemia in the "ischemic penumbra" with electrical failure but sustained energy metabolism and low extracellular potassium and with the possible potential for recovery.[3] The concept of the "ischemic penumbra" of ischemia, tissue with a residual blood flow below a functional blood flow threshold but above the flow threshold for morphological integrity, is of utmost importance for the development of therapeutic regimens for stroke victims.[26] Newer imaging techniques such as MRI and PET performed early and in a serial fashion will be necessary to select cases of infarction with still viable but functionally inactive tissue before we can predictably recommend specific therapy to lessen edema, reverse ischemia, improve microcirculatory failure, and the like.

THERAPY FOR VASCULAR DISEASE

The principles of risk factor management, administration of antiplatelet agents, and serial evaluation watching for symptom recurrence that are recommended in TIA patients are also followed in stroke patients. Surgical management is restricted to patients with very minor strokes, thus limiting the number of invasive angiograms in this group of patients. Angiography is performed in selected cases, including (1) stroke victims under the age of 45 years who fail to demonstrate a clear stroke cause[23]; (2) those who are likely to be heparinized for progressive stroke or progressive basilar artery thrombosis; (3) those with suspected nonatheromatous stroke (i.e., arteritis, fibromuscular dysplasia, dissections); and (4) those with minor stroke and/or TIA who are good surgical candidates.

We reserve anticoagulation administration to patients who have definite cardiac-embolic stroke and/or TIA or occasionally those who fail to have symptom suppression on antiplatelet agents.[7, 12] Because there are improving trends of stroke and MI prevention in patients receiving antiplatelet agents, we choose to use antiplatelet agents rather than warfarin sodium in the majority of our patients. Risk factor management and aggressive rehabilitation programs complement our approach to stroke therapy.

LACUNAR INFARCTION

Case History 3.—A 45-year-old patient with long-standing, poorly controlled hypertension suffers a stroke with findings of face, arm, and leg weakness and no other abnormalities.

DIAGNOSIS, DEFINITION, DIFFERENTIAL

The patient in case 3 has suffered a particularly common type of small infarction known as lacunar stroke. Lacunes are small, deep cerebral infarctions, most often encountered in a setting of hypertension, and refer to the cavity or hole (lacuna) that remains after scavenger cells carry off the infarcted brain tissue.[38] Their location is almost exclusively in the deep regions of the brain, especially the internal capsule, thalamus, basal ganglia, and pons. The importance of lacunae lies in the nature of the clinical syndromes they produce, the opportunities they provide to study cerebral organization, and the special problems they pose in diagnosis and management.[38]

Pathologic studies have demonstrated the occurrence of lacunar infarcts in characteristic locations as a result of small-vessel, arteriolar disease.[36] The typical lacunar syndromes include (1) pure motor hemiparesis with paresis of the face, arm, and leg caused by a lesion in the contralateral internal capsule or basis pontis; (2) pure sensory stroke with paresthesias of arm, leg, and face caused by a lesion in the contralateral thalamus; (3) ataxic hemiparesis with hemiparesis and ipsilateral ataxia caused by a lesion in the contralateral basis pontis or internal capsule; and (4) dysarthria and clumsy hand with hemiataxia and dysarthric speech caused by a lesion in the contralateral basis pontis or internal capsule.

The clinical lacunar syndromes clearly can occur with a variety of vascular and even nonvascular lesions such as intracerebral hematoma, multiple sclerosis, and cerebral metastases. It may also be that emboli and carotid occlusive disease tend to produce larger lacunae with more complex symptomatology.[36] Otherwise, typical lacunae with pure symptomatology are usually thought of as hypertensive patients with small-vessel occlusive disease.

NEURODIAGNOSTIC STUDIES

Because case 3 has typical lacunar findings of pure motor hemiparesis, his neurologic workup centered around a plain CT scan, which was obtained to exclude other pathologic processes. Patients such as this with the triad of a typical lacunar syndrome, hypertension, and either negative results on CT scan (as in case 3) or a CT scan showing a small infarct in the contralateral internal capsule are very likely to have arteriolar end-vessel disease.[36] Usually EEG is normal, because the overlying cerebral cortex remains intact. Carotid Doppler/ultrasound, cerebral angiography and echocardiography do not seem warranted unless the history and clinical examination suggest an atypical presentation. As cases deviate from the triad just mentioned, such as with aphasia or mental changes, the causes of stroke become more diverse, and diagnostic studies must be tailored accordingly.[36, 38]

LACUNAR INFARCT MANAGEMENT DECISIONS

Preventive treatment should involve careful control of hypertension and attention to other risk factors. It also seems reasonable to advise antiplatelet agents in this group of patients combined with observation over time for symptom recurrence or new symptom development.

To date, there is no specific therapy aimed at the area of lacunar infarction itself. Prospective studies on the clinical course of lacunar infarction are also lacking thus far; only after prospective data are available will the efficacy of therapeutic intervention become apparent.[36]

ACUTE HEMORRHAGIC INFARCTION

Case History 4.—A 55-year-old patient suffers a stroke, with findings of headache, confusion, left-sided focal motor seizure activity, left hemiplegia, and left hemisensory loss.

DIAGNOSIS, DEFINITION, DIFFERENTIAL

The patient in case 4 has suffered a hemorrhagic infarction and is showing signs of an irritative mass lesion. Intraparenchymal brain hemorrhages may occur from a variety of causes, the far majority of which are related to hypertensive disease or atherosclerosis. Hemorrhagic infarcts are also more frequent in cerebral embolism, when dissolution of the embolus leaves a necrotic and leaking arterial tree.

The brain's response to this type of space-occupying mass is that of disruption of the normal vascular autoregulation in the region of the hemorrhage combined with rapidly developing cerebral edema, resulting in dramatic increases in intracranial pressure.[45] Lesser degrees of pressure change may account for brief periods of unconsciousness at the moment of hemorrhage; and slower but more persistent changes associated with brain edema and loss of autoregulatory capacity are responsible for the brain herniations and secondary brain stem duret hemorrhages so commonly seen in fatal cases.[45]

Hemorrhagic infarction accounts for about 20% of all strokes in clinical practice. The diagnosis is based on a combination of clinical features, such as severe headache and early alteration in consciousness, and the rapid evolution of events, together with more definitive radiographic procedures. Blood as a cerebral irritant causes early seizure activity and signs of meningeal irritation. Cerebral hemorrhages also are associated with early vasogenic edema formation, often maximal in the first 24–36 hours following the ictus.

While the vast majority of hemorrhagic infarctions are due to hypertensive or atherosclerotic disease, one also has to consider bleeding disorders, traumatic brain hemorrhages, and hemorrhagic conversion of a malignant neoplasm in the differential presentation. In addition, aneurysmal and angiomatous arterial abnormalities are also prone to hemorrhage. To further complicate matters, embolic lesions can convert from ischemic to hemorrhagic foci up to 15% of the time.[7]

NEURODIAGNOSTIC STUDIES

Urgent plain CT or MRI scanning will identify cerebral hemorrhage acutely. Clotted blood, partly due to its calcium content, has a radiographic density in striking contrast to that of the surrounding brain and much greater than that of the fluid-filled ventricular system (Fig 1–7). Therefore, CT scanning allows accurate assessment of the size, situation, and configuration of the hematoma (high density—represented as white on the radiographs), as well as indicating the degree of displacement or distortion of the ventricular system and the presence of any associated edema in the brain parenchyma (diminished density—represented by black or dark gray areas).[45] Contrast-enhancement CT scanning is rarely necessary in the acute stages of a brain hemorrhage and may, in fact, muddle the differential diagnosis in the chronic stages as a result of the overlap in CT scan appearance with brain abscesses and ring-enhancing tumors.

Through a chronological observation of CT images and a histologic observation of experimentally induced brain hemorrhages,[57] we are able to make correlations between the CT scan appearance and the pathologic processes in hemorrhagic infarction. These include (1) acute stage within 4 days after

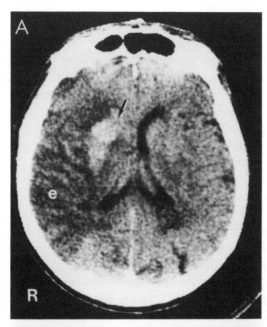

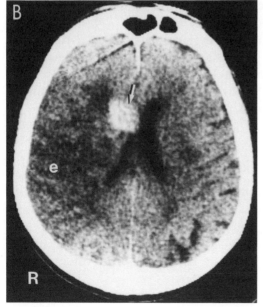

FIG 1–7.
Two levels **(A, B)** of plain CT images on a 59-year-old patient with a hemorrhagic infarct. The hemorrhage *(arrows)* is in the right basal ganglion area with associated cerebral edema (labeled *e*).

hematoma formation—homogeneous high density extending
to the periphery of the lesion, appearance of the necrotic tissue layer; (2) subacute stage between days 5–14 after hematoma formation—decreased density spreading from the periphery and formation of ring enhancement, appearance of
immature connective tissue; and (3) chronic stage starting 15
days after hematoma formation—concentric concentration of
ring enhancement and development of mature connective tissue.[57] We have recently seen the persistence of such chronic
CT changes as late as 4 months following the ictus.[33] The CT
abnormalities prompted a diagnostic brain biopsy and interest-
ingly confirmed the diagnosis of brain hemorrhage.

There is no doubt that CT scanning has revolutionized not
only the ease of diagnosis of hemorrhagic infarction, but has
also provided vital information to formulate a logical treatment
policy.[35] Isotope brain scanning, skull radiographs looking for
pineal gland shift, and lumbar puncture should be performed
urgently if CT is not readily available. Cerebral angiography is
actually preferable to lumbar puncture in lethargic patients
who may already have increased intracranial pressure, because
the lumbar puncture can lead to worsening of mass effect and
potentiate brain herniation. Angiography is most useful in defining aneurysmal or angiomatous causes of hemorrhagic infarction and diagnosing cerebral vasospasm. Angiography may
also reveal neoplastic neovascularity in cases of brain tumor
mimicking stroke.

HEMORRHAGIC INFARCTION: MANAGEMENT DECISIONS

When a diagnosis of hemorrhagic infarction has been established by CT scan, early measures are taken to normalize arterial blood pressure, prevent recurrent hemorrhage, reduce
mass effect, control cerebral edema, and prevent seizures.[41]
Deterioration occurs from cerebral edema, development of
acute hydrocephalus, or rebleeding.

While assessing and providing acute medical stabilization

similar to that for ischemic stroke, a search for bleeding diastheses has to be initiated. Because most hemorrhages appear to have stopped before the patient arrives in the hospital, it has been difficult to assess efforts to stop hemorrhage in the occasional case of continued bleeding.[41] Usually then, administration of agents such as protamine, vitamin K, or fresh frozen plasma are reserved for definite blood dyscrasia diagnoses.

Hypertension has to be controlled, but not overzealously. Because autoregulation is impaired in and around these lesions, significant drops in arterial pressure will produce secondary ischemic damage. There are, however, no clear guidelines available for blood pressure management in acute stroke.[64] We tend to "normalize" blood pressure aggressively in hemorrhagic stroke, hope the pressure is not too low, and urge a careful prospective study in this regard.

Continuous monitoring of intracranial pressure (ICP) may improve the outcome of hemorrhagic infarction and may provide more careful guidelines for arterial blood pressure control.[9] Because the cerebral perfusion pressure (CPP) is determined by the MABP minus the ICP, brain resuscitative therapy can usually be more closely monitored with concomitant measures of blood pressure and ICP using arterial lines and ICP epidural monitors, respectively. Urea, mannitol, and furosemide can be used as cerebral diuretic agents. The stuporous or comatose patient should be intubated to ensure adequate oxygenation and the maintenance of a reduced level of P_{CO_2} at about 25 Hg. Because cerebral edema peaks early and severely in hemorrhagic strokes and because invasive monitoring is often necessary for resuscitative therapy, our hemorrhagic stroke patients are all initially cared for in an intensive care setting. Thus, if ventilatory support becomes necessary, it is also readily available.

Fluid and electrolyte management is also essential because of the common occurrence of inappropriate antidiuretic hormone secretion and because of diuresis induced by agents used for raised levels of ICP. Steroids probably play a small therapeutic role, if any, and are usually not given to our patients. Anticonvulsants are not given unless actual seizures are witnessed.

Most patients undergo serial noncontrast CT scanning to monitor for acute hydrocephalus while hospitalized and, following discharge, are watched for development of delayed hydrocephalus.

Issues of surgical management, treatment of vasospasm, and specific clinical syndromes are not possible in this general review. The reader is referred to one of the excellent reviews available on the subject.[8, 27, 41, 45, 56]

NATURAL HISTORY OF THE DISEASE

IMMEDIATE SURVIVAL

In individual cases, the immediate outlook for life depends on factors such as the age of the patient and the type, size, and anatomical site of the cerebrovascular lesion.[34] Just as the incidence of stroke rises with age, the incidence of fatal stroke is considerably higher in elderly stroke victims. In addition, ischemic strokes carry a much better prognosis than do hemorrhagic ones.

In the Framingham Study,[52] 30-day case fatality rates for initial strokes were 15% for brain infarctions (32/222), 16% for cerebral embolus (10/63), 46% for subarachnoid hemorrhage (18/39), and 82% for intracerebral hemorrhage (14/17). Death in the acute phase occurs mainly from cerebral causes with irreversible failure of vital functions of the brain stem. Death in the subacute and chronic phases occurs primarily from systemic causes such as pneumonia, pulmonary embolus, and ischemic heart disease.

Irrespective of the severity of the stroke, the following proportions of patients under 70 years of age were alive after 5 years: (1) three fourths of those who had neither cardiac symptoms nor blood pressure over 180/100 mm Hg: (2) one half of those in whom only one of these factors was present; and (3) one fourth of those with both cardiac symptoms and hypertension.[34] Thus, the risk of death or recurrence after stroke (about 15% overall) is substantial and profoundly influenced by sex (recurrence rates are double in men) and by cardiac comorbidity and hypertension present prior to the initial stroke.[52]

The vast majority of the initially alert patients, however, survive the acute phase despite stroke subtype. Thus, in patients who are fully alert and who are therefore unlikely to die from the cerebral lesion itself, the prognosis for life depends on the presence or absence of complicating extracerebral disease, in particular cardiac and pulmonary disorders.[2, 34] When a patient has survived the acute phase, we next must assess the chances of recovery of neurologic function.

STROKE MORBIDITY

Although hemorrhagic strokes are much more lethal than ischemic strokes, there is no reason to believe that functional recovery should be less complete after cerebral hemorrhage than after nonhemorrhagic infarction. In fact, in those patients with hemorrhage who are not initially comatose or who have small basal ganglion hemorrhage, recovery is often more complete than in age-matched ischemic patients. Brain hemorrhages certainly exert pressure effects on localized brain regions, but, by spreading tissue layers out instead of necessarily infarcting them, there actually may be less ischemic neuronal compromise than in ischemic lesions. The extent of cerebral damage after arterial occlusion also depends on the availability of collateral blood supply, and this is rarely compromised in primary brain hemorrhages unless by mass effects.

Stroke subtypes with more favorable prognosis for functional recovery include (1) those with a single lacunar infarct; (2) initial ischemic lesions of brain stem; (3) lesions affecting the dominant hemispheric speech centers; and (4) small hemorrhagic strokes without loss of consciousness. Stroke victims with less favorable prognosis for functional recovery include those with (1) persistence of moderate-to-severe hemiparesis or hemiplegia after 1 month without obvious motor improvement; (2) persistent paralysis of conjugate eye movements, especially if combined with hemiplegia and initial impairment of consciousness; (3) persistent hemiflaccidity with motor loss; (4) the presence of homonymous hemianopia with hemiplegia; (5) defects in visuomotor, temporal, and spatial concepts or hemi-inattention; (6) receptive dysphasia; (7) marked mental deterioration, particularly those presenting with urinary incontinence and/or episodes of confusion (multi-infarct dementia); and (8) any combination of these important clinical features.[34]

CONCLUSIONS

Stroke is a leading and worldwide cause of death and disability. While the secular trends for stroke occurrence and mortality are downward, stroke victims are still very prevalent in every medical practice.

All stroke patients deserve hospital admission for diagnosis, but not necessarily for specific medical or surgical therapies; stroke management differs widely, from therapeutic nihilism to enthusiastic treatment with unproved remedies.[25] We urge careful clinical distinction between TIA, completed stroke, and other differential diagnoses, because the management and prognosis vary greatly with the exact diagnosis. Because stroke, apart from being in itself a serious brain disorder, is a more or less incidental manifestation of a steadily progressing generalized vascular disease,[34] our therapeutic zeal reaches a true dichotomy when dealing with stroke victims. It is more than obvious that prevention of stroke or stroke recurrence is the key to reduction of stroke morbidity and mortality. On the other hand, once a stroke has occurred, there may well be no specific medical or surgical intervention we can offer therapeutically other than attempting to delve into the unknowns of unproved or experimental interventions. However, these patients still need restorative nursing and rehabilitation assessment and treatment programs.

We impatiently await future discoveries in the field of stroke diagnosis and management.

ACKNOWLEDGMENTS

Many thanks to Ms. Sue Melvin for her clerical assistance and to Drs. Patrick A. Turski, Charles M. Strother, Lanning W. Houston, Robert E. Polcyn, and Joseph F. Sackett for their advice and radiographic interpretations.

REFERENCES

1. Ackerman RH: Noninvasive diagnosis of carotid disease in the era of digital substraction angiography, in Barnett, HJM (ed): *Neurologic Clinics: Symposium on Cerebrovascular Disease.* Philadelphia, WB Saunders Co, 1983, vol 1.
2. Adams HP, *et al:* The patient with transient ischemic attacks— is this the time for a new therapeutic approach? *Stroke* 1984; 15:371.
3. Astrup J, *et al:* Thresholds in cerebral ischemia—the ischemic penumbra. *Stroke* 1981; 12:723.
4. Barnett HJM: Progress toward stroke prevention: Robert Wartenberg lecture. *Neurology* 1980; 30:1212.
5. Berkoff HA, Levine RL: Management of coronary artery and cerebrovascular disease combinations. *Primary Cardiol.* 1985; 11:74.
6. Candelise L, *et al:* Prognostic significance of hyperglycemia in acute stroke. *Arch Neurol* 1985; 42:661.
7. Cerebral Embolism Task Force: Cardiogenic brain embolism. *Arch Neurol* 1986; 43:71.
8. Chayatte D, Sundt TM: Cerebral vasospasm after subarachnoid hemorrhage. *Mayo Clin. Proc* 1984; 59:498.
9. Duff TA, *et al:* Nonsurgical management of spontaneous intracerebral hematoma. *Neurosurgery* 1981; 9:387.
10. Dyken ML: Anticoagulant and platelet antiaggregating therapy in stroke and threatened stroke, in Barnett HJM (ed): *Neurologic*

Clinics: Symposium on Cerebrovascular Disease. Philadelphia, WB Saunders Co, 1983, vol 1.

11. Dyken ML, *et al:* Risk factors in stroke: A statement for physicians by the subcommittee on risk factors and stroke of the Stroke Council. *Stroke* 1984; 15:1105.

12. Easton JD, and Sherman DG: Management of cerebral embolism of cardiac origin. *Stroke* 1980; 11:433.

13. Fisher CM: Concerning recurrent transient cerebral ischemic attack. *Can Med Assoc J* 1962; 86:1091.

14. Folts JD: Experimental arterial platelet thrombosis, platelet inhibitors, and their possible clinical relevance. *Cardiovasc Rev Rep* 1982, 3:370.

15. Fuster V, Chesebro JH: Series on pharmacology in practice: 10. Antithrombotic therapy: Role of platelet-inhibitor drugs. *Mayo Clin Proc* 1981; 56:102; 185; 265.

16. Futty, DE, *et al:* Cooperative study of hospital frequency and characteristics of transient ischemic attack: V. Symptom analysis. *JAMA* 1977; 238:2386.

17. Gautier JC: Stroke-in-progression. *Stroke* 1985; 16:729.

18. Genton E., *et al:* XIV. Cerebral ischemia: The role of thrombosis and antithrombotic therapy. *Stroke* 1977; 8:150.

19. Grady PA: Pathophysiology of extracranial cerebral arterial stenosis—a critical review. *Stroke* 1984; 15:224.

20. Grotta JC, *et al:* The significance of carotid stenosis or ulceration. *Neurology* 1984; 34:437.

21. Grotta JC, *et al:* Does platelet antiaggregant therapy lessen the severity of stroke? *Neurology* 1985; 35:632.

22. Haas WK: Aspirin for the limping brain, editorial. *Stroke* 1977; 8:299.

23. Hart RG, Miller VT: Cerebral infarction in young adults: A practical approach. *Stroke* 1983; 14:110.

24. Hart RG, Easton JD: Management of cervical bruits and carotid stenosis in preoperative patients. *Stroke* 1983; 14:290.

25. Hachinski V, Norris JW: *The Acute Stroke,* ed 1. Philadelphia, FA Davis Co, 1985.

26. Heiss WD: Flow thresholds of functional and morphological damage of brain tissue. *Stroke* 1983; 14:329.

27. Heros RC, Kistler JP: Intracranial arterial aneurysm—an update. *Stroke* 1983; 14:628.

28. Hornig CR, *et al:* CT contrast enhancement on brain scans and

blood-CSF barrier disturbances in cerebral ischemic infarction. *Stroke* 1985; 16:268.

29. Kannel WB, Wolf PA: epidemiology of cerebrovascular disease, in Ross Russell RW (ed): *Vascular Disease of the Central Nervous System.* Edinburgh, Churchill Livingstone, 1983.
30. Katzman R, *et al:* Brain edema in stroke. *Stroke* 1977; 8:512.
31. Levine RL: The study of cerebral ischemic reversibility: I. A review of positron imaging studies. *Am J Physiol Imag 1986; 1:54–58.*
32. Levine RL, *et al:* The study of cerebral ischemic reversibility: Part II. Fluoromethane positron emission tomographic determination of perfusion reserve in patients with carotid TIA and stroke; preliminary preoperative results. *Am J Physiol Imag* 1986; 1:104–114.
33. Levine RL: Persistent CT changes following an intracerebral hemorrhagic stroke: A case report. *J Neurosurg* (submitted for publication).
34. Marquardsen J: Natural history and prognosis of cerebrovascular disease, in Ross Russell RW (ed): *Vascular Disease of the Central Nervous System.* Edinburgh, Churchill Livingstone, 1983.
35. Meadows JC: Clinical Features of Focal Cerebral Hemisphere Infarction, in Ross Russell RW (ed): *Vascular Disease of the Central Nervous System.* Edinburgh, Churchill Livingstone, 1983.
36. Miller VT: Lacunar stroke: A reassessment. *Arch Neurol* 1983; 40:129.
37. Mohr JP, *et al:* The Harvard Cooperative Stroke Registry: A prospective registry. *Neurology* 1978; 28:754.
38. Mohr JP: Lacunes. *Stroke* 1982; 13:3.
39. Moster ML, *et al:* Chronic subdural hematoma with transient neurological deficits: A review of 15 cases. *Ann Neurol* 1983, 14:539.
40. O'Brien MD: Ischemic cerebral edema: A review. *Stroke* 1979; 10:623.
41. Ojemann RG, Heros RC: Spontaneous brain hemorrhage. *Stroke* 1983; 14:468.
42. Packham MA, Mustard JF: Pharmacology of platelet-affecting drugs. *Circulation* 1980; 62 (suppl V):26.
43. Plum F: What causes infarction in ischemic brain? The Robert Wartenberg Lecture. *Neurology* 1983; 33:222.
44. Powers WJ Raichle ME: Positron emission tomography and its

application to the study of cerebrovascular disease in man. *Stroke* 1985; 16:361.

45. Richardson A: Spontaneous intracerebral hemorrhage, in Ross Russell RW (ed): *Vascular Disease of the Central Nervous System.* Edinburgh, Churchill Livingstone, 1983.

46. Robbins J, *et al:* Acquired neurogenic swallowing problems: Proceedings of clinical and research issues in swallowing and swallowing disorders. NIH Symposium, 1985 (in press).

47. Robertson JT: Carotid endarterectomy, in Barnett HJM (ed): *Neurology Clinics: Symposium on Cerebrovascular Disease.* Philadelphia, WB Saunders Co, 1983, vol 1.

48. Roederer GO, *et al:* The natural history of carotid arterial disease in asymptomatic patients with cervical bruits. *Stroke* 1984; 15:605.

49. Ross RT: Transient tumor attacks. *Arch Neurol* 1983; 40:633.

50. Ross Russell RW: Pathogenesis of transient ischemic attacks, in Barnett HJM (ed): *Neurologic Clinics: Symposium on Cerebrovascular Diseases.* Philadelphia, WB Saunders Co, 1983, vol 1.

51. Ross Russell RW: Transient cerebral ischaemia, in Ross Russell RW (ed): *Vascular Disease of the Central Nervous System.* Edinburgh, Churchill Livingstone, 1983.

52. Sacco RL, *et al:* Survival and recurrence following stroke: The Framingham Study. *Stroke* 1982; 13:290.

53. Sandok RA, *et al:* Guidelines for the management of transient ischemic attacks. *Mayo Clin Proc* 1978; 53:665.

54. Spence JD, Del Maestro RF: Hypertension in acute ischemic strokes. *Arch Neurol* 1985; 42:1000.

55. Spetzler RF, *et al:* Acute NMR changes during MCA occlusion: A preliminary study in primates. *Stroke* 1983; 14:185.

56. Sundt TM, Whisnant JP: Subarachnoid hemorrhage from intracranial aneurysms: Surgical management and natural history of disease. *N Engl J Med* 1978; 299:116.

57. Takasugi S, *et al:* Chronological changes in spontaneous intracerebral hematoma—an experimental and clinical study. *Stroke* 1985; 16:651.

58. Weinfeld FD: The National Survey of Stroke. *Stroke* 1981; 12 (suppl 1):1.

59. Weksler BB, Lewin M: Anticoagulation in cerebral ischemia. *Stroke* 1983; 14:658.

60. Whisnant JP, *et al:* Carotid and vertebral-basilar transient isch-

emic attacks: Effects of anticoagulants, hypertension, and cardiac disorders on survival and stroke occurrence—a population study. *Ann Neurol* 1978; 3:107.

61. Wolf PA, *et al:* Prospective investigations; The Framingham Study and the epidemiology of stroke, in Schoenberg BS (ed): *Advances in Neurology.* New York, Raven Press, 1978, vol 19.

62. Wolf PA, *et al:* Current status of risk factors for stroke, in Barnett HJM (ed): *Neurologic Clincis: Symposium on Cerebrovascular Diseases.* Philadelphia, WB Saunders Co., 1983, vol 1(1).

63. Wood JH, Kee DB: Hemorrheology of the cerebral circulation in stroke. *Stroke* 1985; 16:765.

64. Yatsu FM, Hart RG: Asymptomatic carotid bruit and stenosis: A reappraisal. *Stroke* 1983; 14:301.

65. Ziegler DK: Carotid lesions—to operate or not to operate. *Stroke* 1983; 14:824.

2

The Neuropathology of Stroke

Eleanor F. Branch, Ph.D., P.T.

The familiar clinical picture of stroke, or cerebrovascular accident (CVA), may be defined as the abrupt development of focal neurologic signs and symptoms caused by a pathologic process in a cerebral blood vessel, which results in the destruction of neural tissue. In view of the rarity of cerebral venous and capillary disease, as compared with arterial disease, this discussion will be directed towards the principal affections of cerebral arteries that may lead to stroke.

In general, strokes may be divided into ischemic or hemorrhagic phenomena, although these events may coexist. Ischemic strokes follow the sudden interruption or insufficiency of blood supply to the brain, with resultant infarction. In strokes caused by hemorrhage, on the other hand, while there is a degree of associated tissue destruction, the rapid intracerebral accumulation of blood under arterial pressure may act primarily as an expanding mass lesion, displacing or compressing adjacent brain tissue. In the United States, the majority of CVAs are ischemic in nature. For this reason, the causes and pathologic features of ischemic strokes, as well as several examples of clinical vascular syndromes, will be considered first. Hemorrhagic strokes will be briefly discussed and illustrated in the latter part of this chapter.

ISCHEMIC STROKE

CAUSE

When insufficiency of blood supply to the brain is fleeting, signs and symptoms frequently resolve, and there is little or no pathologic evidence of tissue damage; this has been called transient cerebral ischemia. If the ischemia is prolonged and sufficiently severe, however, infarction of the brain occurs, resulting in the clinical picture of stroke. The term cerebral infarct denotes an area of ischemic necrosis localized to all or part of a particular territory of vascular supply.

Most cerebral infarcts of the arterial tree result from occlusion of a vessel by a thrombus or an embolus.[3] A thrombus most often is secondary to atherosclerosis. Thus, sites of thrombosis tend to be areas where atherosclerosis particularly is prone to develop, such as branching points and sites of curvature of arteries (Fig 2–1). The internal carotid and the basilar arteries, particularly at the origins and terminations of these vessels, are prime sites for atherosclerosis and occlusion.[4] Sites of predilection also include the origins of the common carotid arteries, the proximal parts of the middle cerebral arteries, and the vertebral arteries at their junction to form the basilar artery.[5] In most cases, a cerebral embolus is of cardiac origin and may represent a fragment of thrombus that breaks away from a thrombus on a diseased heart valve, or on the damaged endocardium overlying a myocardial infarction, and enters the circulation (Fig 2–2).[1, 3, 4] Emboli from the heart tend to take a direct route through the carotid system rather than a more winding path through the vertebrobasilar system.[3, 9] Once in an internal carotid artery, in view of its size, an embolus tends to assume a central position in the laminar stream of blood flow and most frequently is carried to the middle cerebral artery—a relatively direct extension of the internal carotid artery—rather than being diverted sharply into more lateral vessels. The embolus comes to rest when its diameter exceeds the caliber of the vessel through which it is moving. Not infrequently, emboli also may arise as fragments of thrombi or of atheromatous material dislodged from atherosclerotic plaques in the aorta or in an internal carotid artery in its course through the neck.[1]

Although it has been emphasized that most ischemic strokes

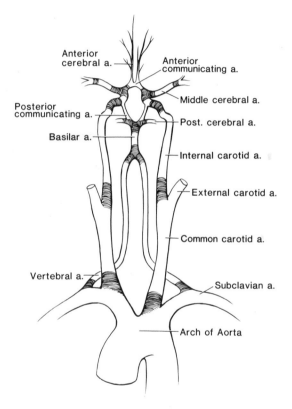

FIG 2–1.
The darkened areas on the diagram illustrate the sites where atherosclerosis is prone to occur in cerebral blood vessels. (Adapted from McDowell FH: Cerebral ischemia and infarction, in Beeson PB, McDermott W, Wyngsarden JB (eds): *Cecil Textbook of Medicine,* ed 15. Philadelphia, WB Saunders Co, 1979; and from Escourolle R, Poirier J, Rubenstein LJ (trans): *Manual of Basic Neuropathology, ed 2.* Philadelphia, WB Saunders Co., 1978.)

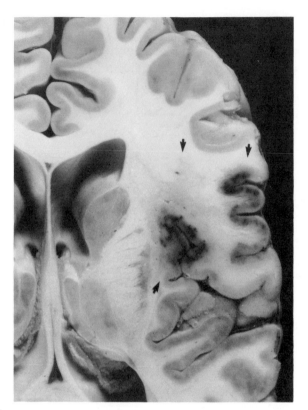

FIG 2–2.
Embolic infarction. A 27-year-old woman suddenly developed numbness and paralysis of the left extremities, associated with temporary unconsciousness and seizures. Death occurred from a pulmonary embolus 2 weeks following stroke. At autopsy, an embolus (believed to have arisen from heart valve vegetations associated with nonbacterial thrombotic endocardosis) was found lodged at the trifurcation of the right middle cerebral artery, with a resultant right frontoparietal infarction. There was softening of the cortex and underlying white matter *(arrows),* with sparing of the basal ganglia. Characteristically, the embolic infarct demonstrated leakage of plasma and red blood cells into the necrotic tissue. (From Burger PC, Vogel FS: *Cerebrovascular Disease.* Teaching Monograph Series, *American Journal of Pathology.* Bethesda, Md, American Association of Pathologists, 1978, p 286. Used by permission.)

are attributable to vascular occlusion caused by atherosclerosis and associated thrombosis or by emboli, other causes include trauma, vascular malformation, infection, neoplasm, and immunologic disorders.[2, 4] It is also of interest that, in a substantial number of cerebral infarcts, examination of the arterial tree fails to reveal any definite structural occlusion.[1, 4] The cause of these infarcts has been variously attributed to factors such as hypotensive episodes, arterial "spasm," and to emboli that have undergone secondary lysis.[9]

There are several hemodynamic factors that influence the appearance and extent of cerebral infarction following occlusion of an arterial vessel[4]; that is, not all occlusions will result in tissue death and clinical signs and symptoms. In addition, as previously noted, infarction may occur in the absence of total vascular occlusion. The hemodynamic factors include the following:

THE PRESENCE AND EFFECTIVENESS OF ANASTOMOTIC CHANNELS

Each cerebral hemisphere is supplied by its own internal carotid artery, which arises from the common carotid. As it emerges from the cavernous sinus, the internal carotid gives off the ophthalmic artery and then, after gaining entrance into the subarachnoid space, bifurcates on the base of the brain into the anterior and middle cerebral arteries (see Fig 2–1). The carotid or "anterior" circulation supplies the optic nerves and retina, the frontal and parietal lobes, and parts of the temporal lobe. A frequently cited anastomotic channel, although suggested by some authors as having limited potential in humans,[3] involves branches of the external carotid artery that join branches of the ophthalmic artery within the orbit (Fig 2–3). Anastomotic connections among cortical branches of the anterior, middle, and posterior cerebral arteries also exist over the surface of the cerebrum.

The two vertebral arteries enter the skull through the foramen magnum. At the pontomedullary junction, these arteries unite to form the basilar artery (Fig 2–4). The vertebral and basilar arteries have three general groups of branches that collectively nourish the medulla, pons, and cerebellum: paramedian, short circumferential, and long circumferential arteries. The basilar artery bifurcates at the level of the midbrain to form the two posterior cerebral arteries, which in turn supply

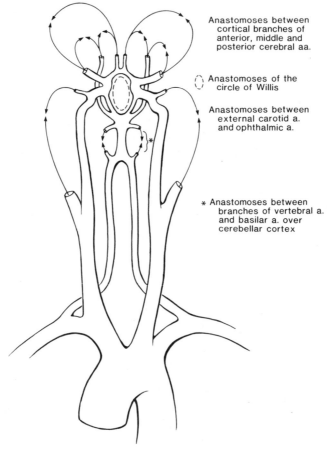

Anastomoses between cortical branches of anterior, middle and posterior cerebral aa.

Anastomoses of the circle of Willis

Anastomoses between external carotid a. and ophthalmic a.

* Anastomoses between branches of vertebral a. and basilar a. over cerebellar cortex

FIG 2–3.
Diagram of the carotid and vertebrobasilar circulations and their chief anastomotic channels (Adapted from Escourolle R, Poirier J, Rubenstein LJ (trans): *Manual of Basic Neuropathology,* ed 2. Philadelphia, WB Saunders Co., 1978.)

the medial portion of the temporal lobe and the occipital lobes. In addition, the vertebrobasilar or "posterior" circulation supplies the midbrain, thalamus, and the inner ear. Tributaries of the vertebral and basilar arteries are sources of anastomotic connections over the surface of the cerebellum (Figs 2–3 and 2–5).

An extremely important anastomotic channel consists of the circle of Willis, which lies at the base of the brain and interconnects the carotid system of one side with that of the other through the anterior communicating artery, and the vertebrobasilar with the carotid system through the posterior communicating arteries (see Fig 2–3). The protective importance of the circle of Willis is illustrated by the fact that the minor deviations from the classic structure of the circle are common,

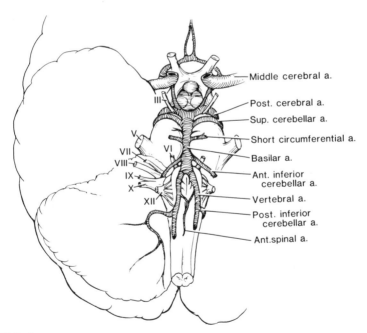

FIG 2–4.
Diagram of the brain stem illustrating major vessels of the vertebrobasilar system; relationships with the carotid system and cranial nerves are shown.

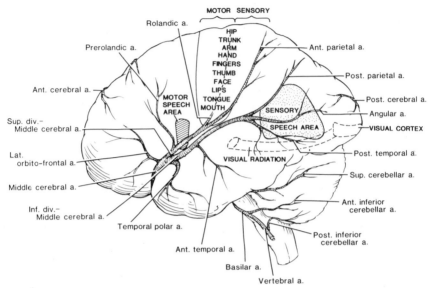

FIG 2–5.
Diagram of the principal arteries on the lateral surfaces of the cerebrum and cerebellum. Note the potential for collateral blood flow between branches of the anterior, middle, and posterior cerebral arteries over the cerebral hemispheres, and the cerebellar arteries over the cerebellum. Some important areas of cerebral localization also are shown.

but are frequently innocuous in the absence of occlusive disease; however, when part of the vascular supply to the brain is compromised, they can become functionally significant by reducing an opportunity for collateral flow (Figs 2–6 and 2–7).[3]

These and other anastomotic networks protect the brain by allowing for alternative routes that can circumvent obstruction of any of the main arteries supplying the brain (see Fig 2–3). For example, obstruction in an internal carotid artery in the neck, extracranially, may be bypassed through anastomotic channels between the external carotid artery and the ophthalmic artery, such that blood flows in retrograde fashion through the ophthalmic artery into the internal carotid within the cranium. In this situation, collateral flow may also occur through the vertebrobasilar system and the opposite internal carotid artery, by way of the anterior communicating artery. In another example, obstruction in a vertebral artery might be bypassed through channels connecting the posterior inferior cerebellar artery (a branch of the vertebral artery) with the anterior inferior cerebellar artery (a branch of the basilar artery) on the surface of the cerebellum (see Figs 2–3 and 2–5). A third example involves the circle of Willis directly. Occlusion of one anterior cerebral artery, proximal to the anterior communicating artery, might not cause symptoms and

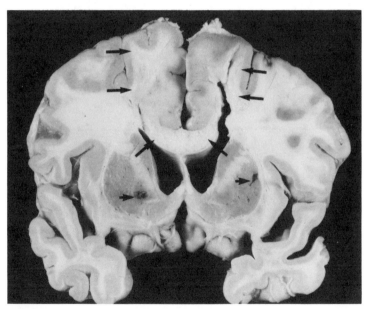

FIG 2–6.
Cerebral infarction associated with an anomaly of the circle of Willis. A 78-year-old hypertensive man died of pneumonia 3 weeks after the onset of dizziness, aphasia, bilateral lower extremity weakness, right upper extremity paresthesias, and urinary incontinence. At autopsy, there was an infarct in the distribution of both anterior cerebral arteries including the corpus callosum *(long arrows)* as well as marked atherosclerosis of the cerebral vessels. Lacunar infarcts were present in the basal ganglia *(short arrows).*

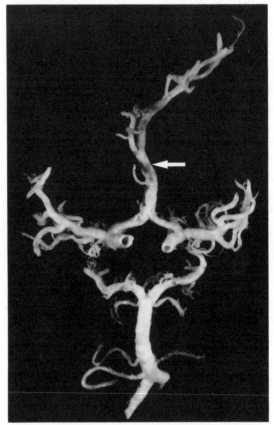

FIG 2–7.
Striking anomaly of the circle of Willis. The anterior cerebral arteries of the patient described in Figure 2–6 had a common trunk for 3 cm before dividing into the right and left anterior cerebral arteries. The distal centimeter of the anterior cerebral artery trunk was darkened *(arrow)* and, on cut section, was found to be completely occluded by a thrombus.

signs because the contralateral carotid system could supply blood to the anterior cerebral artery distal to the occlusion through the intact anterior communicating artery. Cortical anastomoses might be of some benefit as well.

In spite of these and other anastomotic connections, anatomical arrangements vary from individual to individual (see Fig 2–7). In addition, the channels themselves may be occluded by atherosclerosis and therefore may be ineffective in preventing infarction.[4]

SITE OF OCCLUSION

Occlusion of a proximal blood vessel such as the internal carotid artery, as a result of anastomotic channels, may produce a limited pathologic lesion and minor clinical signs and symptoms. However, should the arterial substitution network be anatomically absent or occluded, the infarct may then be massive and may involve the entire arterial territory. In arterial occlusion involving a distal vessel such as a branch of the middle cerebral artery, the anastomotic possibilities are limited to the arterial network over the cortical surface; these anastomoses are generally ineffective in preventing infarction, although the area of tissue death will be limited in extent.[4, 6, 8]

TYPE OF OCCLUSION

In general, thrombosis leading to gradual occlusion will facilitate the development of an anastomotic network. The resulting infarct may then be relatively limited in extent. By contrast, emboli produce sudden occlusion, following which reirrigation of the tissue may be inadequate; hence, the resulting infarct is usually extensive.[1] However, if the embolus is lysed rapidly, blood flow may be reestablished in time to prevent such extensive damage.

GROSS AND MICROSCOPIC FEATURES OF CEREBRAL INFARCTION

Acute arterial occlusion of sufficent duration produces tissue death within minutes, but gross and histologic changes are not apparent for 12–24 hours.[3] By 24–36 hours, the damaged zone appears grossly as a soft, edematous, expansile lesion that obscures the usually distinct junction between white and gray matter (Fig 2–8). In the case of thrombotic occlusion, vascular congestion within the lesion may be present, imparting a dusky discoloration to the tissue. Embolic infarcts characteristically show leakage of plasma and red blood cells into the necrotic tissue (see Fig 2–2). Edema is usually inconsequential in small lesions, but may be life-threatening in large infarcts because of the potential for producing transtentorial herniation of the brain with resultant brain stem compression (Fig 2–9).

From 2–10 days, the edema persists, but to a decreasing extent, while the boundaries between the infarcted area and adjacent viable tissue gradually become better defined (Fig 2–10). Coincident with this, a process of liquefaction and cavitation begins, by which a solid infarct over weeks or months is converted into a cyst (Figs 2–11 to 2–13). This changing appearance of a cerebral infarct is largely a result of the activity of macrophages responding to the presence of necrotic tissue[3] and, in addition, is reflective of the fact that repair cannot occur by neuronal replication. Unlike the acute expansile lesion, an old infarct retracts, and, when the tissue involved is on the cortical surface, the depressed area is covered on its border by a meningeal membrane (see Figs 2–10 and 2–11).

Microscopically, by the end of the first day, the neurons within the infarcted area show signs of ischemic damage, including contraction of the cell body, disappearance of the Nissl substance, and shrinkage and increased staining of the nucleus. Oligodendrocytes are next to neurons in vulnerability to ischemia, and usually they disappear rapidly in the area of infarction. In addition, myelin structures lose their usual affinity for stains, and vascular congestion is apparent. Between 24–48 hours, there is evidence of phagocytic activity in the area; neutrophilic leukocytes becomes prominent in the infarct. This type of cellular exudation is of brief duration, and after 48 hours neutrophils are replaced by macrophages, whose function over time is to clean up the necrotic debris

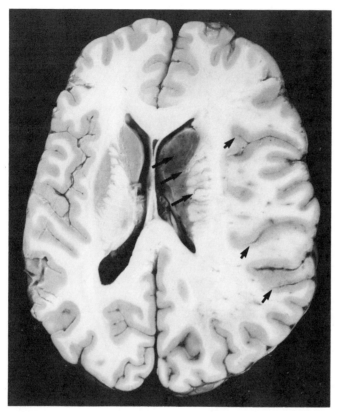

FIG 2–8.
Cerebral infarct of 2 days' duration, with transtentorial herniation. This 59-year-old hypertensive woman suddenly developed sensory and motor deficits of the left extremities and face, and hemianopsia, but was alert and oriented. Sixteen hours later she became unresponsive and developed clinical signs of tentorial herniation. At autopsy, the mildly atherosclerotic right internal carotid was occluded by a fresh thrombus. The right cerebral hemisphere was softened and markedly swollen, and displaced the ventricular system. The infarction in the distribution of the middle cerebral artery is difficult to distinguish (compare with Figs 2–11 and 2–12), but obscuring of the gray-white junction can be appreciated *(short arrows).* The caudate, putamen, globus pallidus, and internal capsule also show ischemic damage *(long arrows).* (From Burger PC, Vogel FS: *Cerebrovascular Disease.* Teaching Monograph Series, *American Journal of Pathology.* Bethesda, Md, American Association of Pathologists, 1978, p 286. Used by permission.)

(Fig 2–14, *A-E*).[3, 10] When laden with debris, these macrophages (called "gitter cells") migrate to blood vessels and slip through the vessel walls to gain access to the bloodstream. Many of these macrophages originate as blood-borne monocytes that leave the bloodstream in response to tissue necrosis;

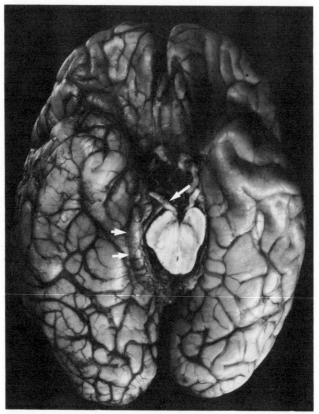

FIG 2–9.
Same patient as in Fig 2–8. Acute expansion of the brain displaced medial temporal lobe over edge of tentorium *(short arrows),* and the right third nerve *(long arrow)* was contused. Death occurred from ischemia and hemorrhage in the brain stem, secondary to herniation. (From Burger PC, Vogel FS: *Cerebrovascular Disease.* Teaching Monograph Series, *American Journal of Pathology.* Bethesda, Md, American Association of Pathologists, 1978, p 286. Used by permission.)

another source of these macrophages is believed to be elements indigenous to the brain, the microglia. Proliferation of capillary endothelial cells can be observed as early as 4 days and is a prominent feature by several weeks (Figs 2–14, *A* and *B*). By 48 hours, astrocytes, which are more resistant to isch-

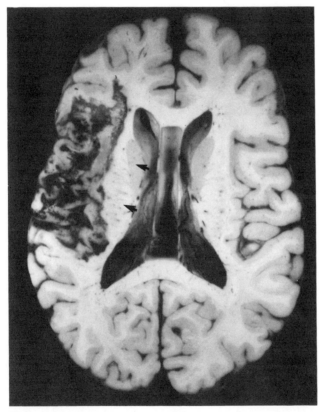

FIG 2–10.
Cerebral infarct of 3 weeks' duration. An infarct in the distribution of the left middle cerebral artery, in a 45-year-old man, was accompanied by right hemiplegia and aphasia. The boundaries between the necrotic area and adjacent viable tissue are better defined than in the lesion described in Figure 2–8, and edema is not obvious. A thromboembolus was present at the trifurcation of the left middle cerebral artery, distal to the penetrating branches that supply parts of the basal ganglia and internal capsule; the latter structures *(arrows),* therefore, are not in the territory of infarction.

emia than are neurons and oligodendrocytes, begin to prolif-
erate and hypertrophy at the edge of the lesion. Their processes assume a tangled pattern, and it is these processes that
gradually form the typical glial scar surrounding the infarcted
area (Fig 2–14, *D* and *F*). This type of scarring is unlike that

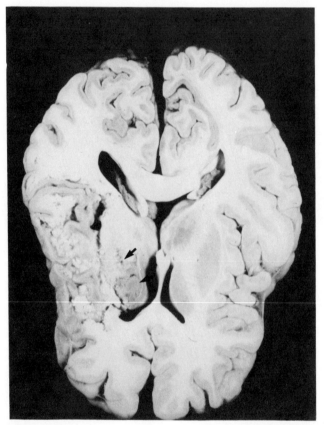

FIG 2–11.
Cerebral infarct of 6 weeks' duration. An infarct in the distribution of the
right middle cerebral artery shows marked liquefaction and beginning of
cavitation. At autopsy, this 49-year-old man, with a history of myocardial
infarction and congestive heart failure, had multiple mural thrombi in the
heart; an embolus (though not demonstrable) was considered as a possible cause of this lesion. In contrast to Figure 2–10, this infarct includes
parts of the basal ganglia and internal capsule *(arrows).*

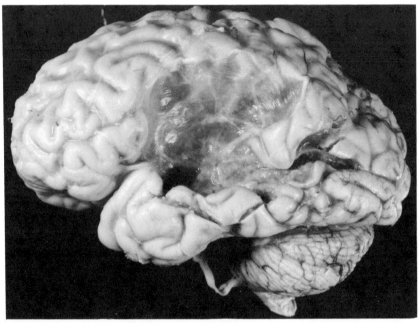

FIG 2–12.
Cerebral infarct of 4 years' duration, lateral view. Four years prior to his death, this 62-year-old man developed a right hemiparesis and aphasia. At autopsy, there was approximately 90% occlusion of the left internal carotid artery by atherosclerosis. The retracted and cavitated lesion is typical of old cerebral infarctions and, in this case, defines the cortical distribution of the left middle cerebral artery. In the lateral view, the meningeal membranes covering the cystic area are well appreciated.

seen in other areas of the body, where the production of collagen by fibroblasts is the mechanism of scar formation. In its final form, the cystic cavity is surrounded by a glial scar, filled with a clear fluid, and traversed by vascular trabeculae; a few residual gitter cells may be present (see Fig 2–14, *E*). In the case of large infarcts, 10 or more years may be required for this stage to be reached.[10] When examined microscopically, older infarcts may show preservation of the subpial cortex (see Fig 2–14, *C*), where neurons have been replaced by astrocytes. It has been suggested that this region is supplied by nu-

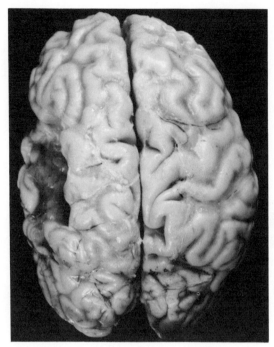

FIG 2–13.
Same patient as in Fig 2–12, superior view.

trients and oxygen that diffuse from the cerebrospinal fluid; the more resistant astrocytes are able to survive in such an environment.

A summary of the previously discussed gross and microscopic features of cerebral infarction is presented in Table 2–1.

CLINICAL VASCULAR SYNDROMES

Occlusion of individual cerebral arteries by a thrombus or embolus produces syndromes that are characteristic for each artery.[7] A knowledge of these syndromes is frequently useful in making the differential diagnosis between cerebrovascular diseases and other disorders of the brain. Although the correlation between the vascular anatomy and the signs and symp-

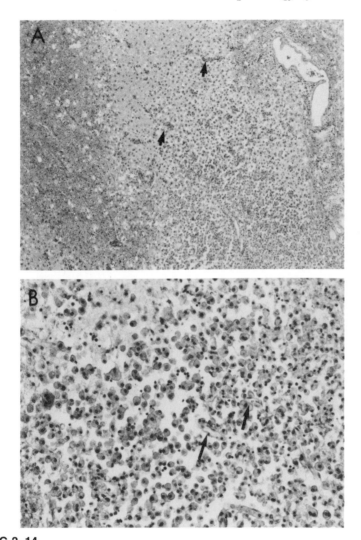

FIG 2–14.
Microscopic features of cerebral infarction. **A,** Infarct in the white matter of
the cerebral cortex, 2 weeks duration. The middle of the field contains necrotic tissue, reactive macrophages, and proliferating capillaries *(arrows).*
At the left border is an area of edematous white matter with distended
(ballooned) myelin sheaths (×52). **B,** A mass of macrophages ("gitter
cells") engulfing necrotic debris (granular material in the background), in a
2-week-old infarct. Proliferating capillaries also can be seen *(arrows)*
(×170). *(Continued.)*

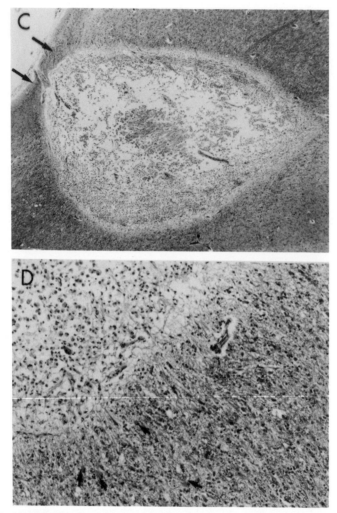

FIG 2–14 (cont.).
C, Four-month-old infarct. Note sparing of the subpial cortex *(arrows)*. The cavitated nature of the lesion is obvious. Necrotic debris, being removed by macrophages, can be seen in the center of the cyst; vascular trabeculae are also present (×25). **D,** Proliferating astrocytes *(arrows)* around the periphery of a 4-month-old infarct. Their processes assume a tangled pattern characteristic of a glial scar. At the upper left of the field, macrophages are still present in the infarct, removing necrotic debris (×130). *(Continued.)*

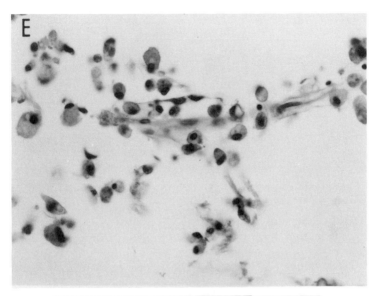

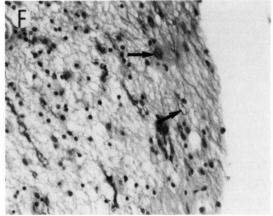

FIG 2–14 (cont.).
E, The cavity of this year-old infarct still contains some gitter cells and strands of blood vessels (×400). **F,** Four-year-old cortical infarct. Hypertrophied astrocytes *(arrows)* and their processes have woven a glial scar at the edge of the cystic cavity on the right (×250).

toms demonstrated by the patient is far from perfect, because of the factors that may modify the extent of ischemic damage (e.g., anastomotic channels), a few examples of these syndromes are warranted.

THE MIDDLE CEREBRAL ARTERY SYNDROME

Infarction in the territory of the middle cerebral artery underlies the most common stroke syndrome.[2] This artery supplies most of the cortex and white matter of the convexity of the cerebral hemisphere, including the frontal, parietal, and parts of the temporal lobes (see Fig 2–5); in addition, small penetrating branches, given off soon after the origin of the middle cerebral artery from the internal carotid artery, supply parts of the internal capsule and basal ganglia. Thrombus formation or embolism is more common in one or more of the cortical branches of the artery than the main trunk itself.[4, 7] Occlusion of the latter produces extensive neurologic disturbance, with profound contralateral hemiplegia and sensory loss, homonymous hemianopsia, and, depending on the hemisphere involved, either language disturbance or impaired spatial perception; the individual may be rendered stuporous if the infarct is massive. On the other hand, when individual cortical branches are occluded, only fragments of the syndrome appear, such as agnosia, hemianopsia, hemiplegia, or dysphasia.

In middle cerebral artery infarcts, weakness and sensory loss characteristically affect the face and arm more than the leg. This is because the face and arm representation is on the convexity of the motor and sensory strips (see Fig 2–5), whereas the leg resides on the medial surface of the hemisphere, and the latter area of the brain is supplied by the anterior cerebral artery (see Fig 2–6). Motor weakness and sensory impairment are greatest in the hands, because the more proximal limbs and trunk tend to have greater representation in both hemispheres. Paraspinal muscles, for example, are rarely weak in unilateral cerebral lesions in the distribution of middle cerebral artery. Similarly, the facial muscles of the forehead and

TABLE 2–1.
Summary of Gross and Microscopic Features of Cerebral Infarction

TIME FOLLOWING ISCHEMIC EVENT	GROSS FEATURES	MICROSCOPIC FEATURES
<12 hours	No visible changes	No visible change
24–48 hours	Area soft, edematous, expansile; gray-white junction indistinct	Myelin pale, neutrophilic exudate, neuronal damage
48 hours–10 days	Infarct boundary better defined	Macrophages prominent, beginning proliferation of capillaries & astrocytes
10 days	Liquefaction begins	Marked macrophage proliferation, continued removal of necrotic debris
>1 month	Progressive conversion of infarct into cystic cavity	Continued macrophage activity, marked astrocyte proliferation surrounding fluid-filled cyst

muscles of the pharynx and jaw are respresented bilaterally in the hemispheres, and, therefore, are usually spared. Muscle tone usually is decreased initially, but gradually increases over days and weeks to spasticity. Sensory loss tends to involve discriminative and proprioceptive modalities more than pain and temperature, which may be impaired but usually are not lost. Joint position, two-point discrimination, and tactile localization may all be diminished or absent. Visual field impairment is a result of damage to the optic radiation to the cortex (see Fig 2–5). If the lesions are in the dominant hemisphere, aphasia, apraxia, or agnosia may be demonstrated. Infarction of the right hemispheric convexity, especially the parietal lobe, tends to cause disturbances of spatial perception; there may be difficulty in copying simple pictures or diagrams, in finding one's way about, or in putting on one's clothes properly. Awareness of space and the patient's own body contralateral to the lesion may be particularly affected. The patient may deny that his affected limbs are paralyzed (anosognosia) when there is an obvious hemiplegia. Such phenomena may occur independently of visual field defects.

THE POSTERIOR INFERIOR CEREBELLAR ARTERY SYNDROME

As an aid in understanding the syndromes of vertebrobasilar origin, each side of the brain stem can be divided into two parts, the paramedian and the lateral.[7] The paramedian areas are nourished by short vessels from the vertebral and basilar arteries at various levels of the brain stem. The lateral areas are supplied by vessels that travel some distance from their point of origin before entering the brain stem (short and long circumferential arteries); branches from these latter vessels also supply the cerebellum (see Figs 2–4 and 2–5).

Let us first consider the paramedian area. Because the important structures in this area of the brain stem are the motor nuclei of the third, fourth, sixth, and twelfth cranial nerves, the corticospinal tract, and the medial lemniscus, the syndromes that result from occlusions of these vessels will consist of a paralysis of one or more cranial nerves on the same side of the body as the lesion, and varying degrees of impairment of sensation and loss of motor function of the arm and leg on the contralateral side. Depending on the extent of infarction, bilateral signs may be present, such as quadriparesis, disturbance in consciousness, and gaze and pupillary disturbances. Such signs and symptoms also accompany occlusion of the basilar artery itself.

Occlusion of one of the long circumferential vessels that supply the lateral areas of the brain stem will cause symptoms of dysfunction of the cerebellum and of the nuclei and tracts in the lateral portion of the brain stem. The important structures in the latter are the motor nuclei of the fifth, seventh, and tenth cranial nerves; the sensory nuclei of the fifth and eighth cranial nerves; the descending sympathetic pathways; and the spinothalamic tract. Three important arteries nourish these areas: the posterior inferior cerebellar artery, a branch of the vertebral artery, supplies the lateral area in the caudal portion of the brain stem (see Figs 2–4 and 2–5); the anterior inferior cerebellar artery, a branch of the basilar artery, supplies the lateral area of the brain stem in the region of the pons; and the lateral area of the upper portion of the brain stem is supplied by the superior cerebellar artery, also a branch of the basilar artery.

Infarction in the distribution of the posterior inferior cerebellar artery occurs more frequently than of any other cerebellar artery.[9] The signs and symptoms that result in this syndrome, called Wallenberg's syndrome, are (1) dysphagia and dysarthria resulting from weakness of the homolateral muscles of the palate (nucleus ambiguus of the tenth nerve); (2) impairment of pain and temperature sense of the homolateral side of the face (descending root and tract of the trigeminal nerve); (3) Horner's syndrome on the side of the lesion (descending sympathetic fibers); (4) nystagmus (vestibular nuclei); (5) cerebellar dysfunction in the homolateral arm and leg (the inferior cerebellar peduncle and cerebellum); and (6) impairment of pain and thermal sense over the opposite arm and leg (spinothalamic tract). In view of the fact that the infarction occurs in the lateral area of the medulla, this syndrome has been called the lateral medullary plate syndrome.

In conclusion, although it is generally possible to designate the involvement of a particular artery on the basis of the clinical picture presented by the patient, it should be remembered that anatomical and physiologic differences among patients may alter the clinical presentation; "pure" syndromes may not be seen.

HEMORRHAGIC STROKE

Hemorrhagic strokes most commonly are sequelae of rupture of intracerebral arteries, associated with hypertension.[3] Not infrequently, arterial bleeding into the brain parenchyma results in such a rapid accumulation of blood that, not only are focal neurologic deficits produced, but, more significantly for the patient, the concomitant rise in intracranial pressure results in lethal transtentorial or foraminal herniation. Such a hematoma may also rupture into the ventricular system with fatal consequences, largely as the result of compression of vital

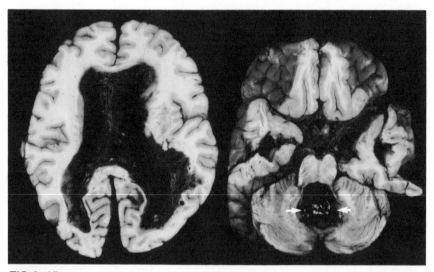

FIG 2–15.
Fatal intracerebral hemorrhage. A 38-year-old man was found unresponsive, taken to the hospital, and died shortly thereafter. There was no history of trauma. At autopsy, there was expansion of the left cerebral hemisphere, mild tentorial herniation, and extensive subarachnoid hemorrhage. When the brain was sectioned, the entire ventricular system was found to be filled with a cast of blood; the fourth ventricle was particularly distended *(arrows)*. A potential site for the hemorrhage was found in the thalamus, but no abnormal vessels were identified. Although the patient did not have a documented history of hypertension, multiple small lacunar infarcts, as well as hypertensive changes in small blood vessels, were noted in the brain; therefore, the occurrence of the fatal hemorrhage was attributed to hypertension.

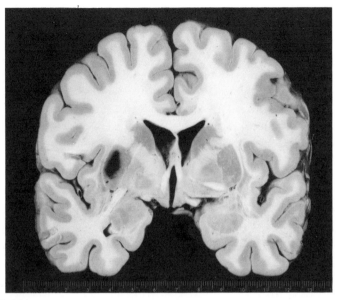

FIG 2–16.
Recent, localized, intracerebral hypertensive hemorrhage. This 58-year-old man had a 12-year history of poorly controlled hypertension and chronic renal failure. Three weeks before his death, he was admitted to the hospital with headache, nausea, vomiting, lethargy, and confusion, compatible with the diagnosis of hypertensive encephalopathy. Except for the lethargy and confusion, and a left central facial paresis, he appeared neurologically intact at that time (the family gave a history of slurring of speech 4 months before). At autopsy, this focus of hemorrhage in the right putamen measured 1 × 0.5 × 0.5 cm and was considered to be several months old.

medullary centers as the fourth ventricle is distended with blood (Fig 2–15). Less frequently, bleeding is not as extensive, only focal signs and symptoms may result, and the patient survives the incident (Fig 2–16). In such cases, recovery of function may be better than that following an ischemic event, because hemorrhage often damages to a greater extent by displacement and compression of tissue than by tissue destruction.[1]

The repair process following a hemorrhagic event is similar to that seen in ischemic strokes, with the ultimate production of a cyst. When tissue destruction is minimal, a hemosiderin-stained slit may be all that marks the site of the former hemorrhage, although many months may be required for the extravasated blood to be removed.

Approximately 80% of hypertensive hemorrhages are situated in the cerebral hemispheres. Among these, the majority are in the basal ganglia-thalamus.[3] The remaining 20% predominantly are found in the pons and cerebellum. The nature of the underlying vascular lesion that leads to arterial rupture is poorly understood. Microaneurysms of smaller arteries and arterioles (Charcot-Bouchard aneurysms), resulting from degenerative changes associated with long-standing hypertension, have been implicated in the pathogenesis of the disorder[3]; however, in a number of cases such aneurysms have not been identified at autopsy.[8] Another contributing factor may be hemorrhage into small infarcts (referred to as "lacunae"), which are frequent findings in the basal ganglia, thalamus, and pons of patients with arteriosclerotic changes in small cerebral arteries, particularly in the setting of hypertension (see Fig 2–6).[3]

CONCLUSION

The preceding illustrated review of the salient etiologic and pathologic features of ischemic and hemorrhagic strokes has been designed to provide the reader with an appreciation of the factors that may help to explain the variability of signs and symptoms with which stroke patients present. As we have seen, even patients with occlusions of identical arteries clinically may appear quite different, for a variety of hemodynamic reasons. In addition, the extensive residual loss of brain tissue, which at times may be associated with a stroke, has been demonstrated.

REFERENCES

1. Ad Hoc Committee, Advisory Council for the National Institute of Neurological Disease and Blindness: *A Classification and Outline of Cerebrovascular Diseases.* Public Health Service, Reprinted from *Neurology* May 1958; 8:1–34.

2. Brust JCM: Stroke: Diagnostic, anatomical, and physiological considerations, in Kandel ER, Schwartz JH (eds): *Principles of Neural Science*. New York, Elsevier/North-Holland, 1981, pp 667–679.

3. Burger PC, Vogel FS: *Cerebrovascular Disease*. Teaching Monograph Series, *The American Journal of Pathology*. Bethesda, Md, The American Association of Pathologists, 1978.

4. Escourolle R, Poirier J, Rubinstein LJ (trans): *Manual of Basic Neuropathology*, ed 2. Philadelphia, WB Saunders Co, 1978.

5. McDowell FH: Cerebral ischemia and infarction, in Beeson PB, McDermott W, Wyngaarden JB (eds): *Cecil Textbook of Medicine*, ed 15. Philadelphia, WB Saunders Co, 1979, pp 778–794.

6. McMenemey WH, Smith WT: The central nervous system, in Symmers W St C (ed): *Systemic Pathology*, ed 2. New York, Churchill Livingstone, 1979, vol 5, pp 2170–2183.

7. Merritt HH: *A Textbook of Neurology*, ed 6. Philadelphia, Lea & Febiger, 1979.

8. Raichle ME, DeVivo DC, Hanaway J: Disorders of cerebral circulation, in Eliasson SG, Prensky AL, Hardin WB Jr (eds): *Neurological Pathophysiology*, ed 2. New York, Oxford University Press, 1978, pp 278–304.

9. Toole JF: *Cerebrovascular Disorders*, ed. 3. New York, Raven Press, 1984.

10. Weller RO: *Color Atlas of Neuropathology*. New York, Oxford University Press, 1984.

3

Recovery From Stroke

Paul Bach-y-Rita, M.D.
Richard Balliet, Ph.D.

Recovery from stroke can be considered to be divisible into "spontaneous" recovery and recovery obtainable by interventions that influence neural mechanisms. The emphasis in this chapter will be on the latter category. The neuroanatomical, neurophysiological, and neuropharmacological bases of recovery from brain damage and the role of environmental factors will be discussed. Finally, the development and evaluation of some rehabilitation methodologies, primarily those related to late recovery, will be examined.

SPONTANEOUS RECOVERY

The stages of recovery have been described by several authors, including Twitchell[68] and Brunnstrom[17] and have been reviewed elsewhere.[7] In the human studies, it may be difficult to determine the spontaneous recovery, since most patients get at least some passive ranging. However, in primate studies, Travis and Woolsey[67] have demonstrated the importance of physical therapy in avoiding contractures that would mask the spontaneous recovery; they provided passive limb, trunk, and neck movements 10–14 times per day in their brain-lesioned monkeys until the animals could get along by themselves.

Thus, they were able to demonstrate considerable return of function following extensive neocortical damage. As a result of this therapy, a totally decorticated monkey learned to right itself, get to its feet unaided, sit, stand, and walk alone. Results such as these had not been obtained in previous studies that had not included therapy.

FACTORS RELEVANT TO RECOVERY OBTAINABLE BY INTERVENTIONS

NEURAL MECHANISMS

An analysis of the neural mechanisms involved in the damage and the recovery process should lead to improved therapy methodologies. Three categories will be discussed here: neuroanatomical, neurophysiological, and neurotransmitter considerations.

NEUROANATOMICAL CONSIDERATIONS

Hierarchical Organization of the Brain.—Phylogenetically and ontogenetically, the nervous system develops in a hierarchical sequence. The entire central nervous system (CNS) can be divided into the archi-, the paleo-, and the neomammalian parts. The archi component is the central core and includes the autonomic and reticular systems of the neuraxis and the archi cerebellovestibular system. The paleomammalian part includes the protopathic or protective systems, while the neomammalian portion represents the epicritic or exploratory component of the CNS. The majority of the neuronal processes projecting from the archi systems do so bilaterally and are highly multisynaptic in character. The pathways of the paleo system tend to cross (decussate) and exert their major influences contralaterally and have fewer multisynaptic connections. The neocerebral systems appear to give humans laterality: they have the most direct fiber systems between lower and higher centers and vice versa, and are the last to develop full functional capabilities, often years after birth. The neocortical structures that constitute 90% of the human brain mass are also the most subject to damage because of their exposed location and the fact that the blood vessels supplying these structures are principally terminal branches, thus allowing little opportunity for collateral circulation.[53]

The phylogenetically older levels of the CNS continually set and reset the background chemical, emotional, and muscular tone, including balance and timing, that is necessary for normal stereofunctioning, learning, and manipulating the three-dimensional environment. The nuclear centers and fiber projections of all three systems (archi, paleo, and neo) synapse with commissural interneurons so that the bilaterality of the brain is preserved, in spite of the evolutionary trend towards lateralization of function. Thus, even "hemiplegic" patients (with unilateral brain damage) reveal at least some bilateral dysfunction.[53]

Integrative Structures.—Throughout vertebrate phylogeny, the motor systems undergo fewer changes than the sensory systems. Basically, the motor systems either respond or do not respond, depending on the integrity of the sensory systems coupled with the integrative action of the CNS. Only a few reflexes in man (e.g., myotatic, such as the patellar reflex) are simple two-neuron reflexes. The rest are more complex, including feedback circuits, ascending and descending collaterals, and commissural interneuronal connections. In most cases, thousands of neurons are involved in regulating the activity of a single cell. Almost all the ascending and descending fibers in the CNS white matter are long interneurons. For example, the majority of the pyramidal tract fibers are interneurons with integrative functions. Some synapse on other interneurons before synapsing on alpha and gamma motoneurons, while many are concerned with modifying incoming sensory information and/or relaying information to subcortical nuclear areas including the cerebellum. Most pathways (the very recent less so) have numerous collaterals projecting to adjacent nuclear areas of the neuraxis, and the numbers of commissural neurons (which at all levels of the body transmit information from one side to the other) increase as the phylogenetic scale is ascended. These commissural interneurons play a role in bilateral coordination and are particularly important since most human activities (e.g., dressing) are bilateral.[53]

Ipsilateral Pathways.—Each half of the brain primarily controls movement on the opposite side of the body. However, in addition to contralateral control, the brain also demonstrates ipsilateral control. This is quite apparent in hemispherectomy cases. For example, Gardner[32] showed that a considerable amount of motor control, including walking, returned in a patient following removal of a hemisphere (520 gm of tissue!). Glees[34] reviewed animal and clinical hemispherectomy studies and pointed out that intellectual function and sensory and motor control for the whole body could be subserved by the remaining hemisphere. Although far from complete, the recovery was sufficient in some cases to allow bimanual function.

Brodal,[14] in an analysis of his recovery from a stroke, emphasized the ipsilateral defects that are not usually described in a clinical examination because they are not looked for. The ipsilateral deficits have been documented by several research groups. Jebson et al.[42] noted that function of the "normal" hand revealed deficits in right and left hemiplegic patients, with the most significant findings being slowness of writing, eating, and emptying and filling cans. McClanahan and Vigano[48] studied an early (less than 2 months) and late (more than 1 year) group of patients with right hemisphere lesions and demonstrated significant deficits in two gross motor tests requiring proximal limb speed and coordination: hand-arm tap and directed reaching, while fine motor tests showed few differences from controls. Most of the patients were unaware of the ipsilateral deficits. McClanahan and Vigano[48] discussed their findings in terms of the anatomical data revealing ipsilateral control of proximal limb muscles. Brinkman and Kuypers,[13] summarizing their work and the work of others, found that each half of the brain has full control over arm, hand, and finger movements contralaterally, but mainly controls relatively proximal arm movements ipsilaterally. While Mc-Clanahan and Vigano[48] did not find differences between patient groups and controls in two-point discrimination or sharp-dull sensory tests, they suggested that since the gross motor tests have a component of directed reaching and a perception of the relationship of body to objects, parietal cortex dysfunction could have contributed to the functional deficits. Similarly, Mountcastle et al.[54] have described parietal cortex cells that were active only during reaching within the immediate extrapersonal space, and have shown that some of them are related to ipsilateral arm movements.

NEUROPHYSIOLOGICAL CONSIDERATIONS

Neurophysiological data related to recovery from stroke has been discussed extensively elsewhere (e.g., Bach-y-Rita[3–7]), and so only a few points will be presented here.

Inhibitory Mechanisms.—The development of rehabilitation is closely related to selective function (and to the precise coordinated movements that are disturbed by a brain lesion). For example, a child learning to write initially demonstrates electromyographic (EMG) activity in virtually all the muscles related to the hand. As ability increases, there is a progressive reduction of muscle activity until the stage where there is a minimum of activity, coordinated to produce just the motor control necessary for writing, which is relatively fatigue-free.[57] Similarly, reflexes that are normal shortly after birth (e.g., Babinski) are inhibited, and reappear only following brain damage.

Inhibition is much more important than is generally appreciated: much of what is taught emphasizes excitation while virtually ignoring inhibition. Even the concept of "synaptic facilitation" has been seriously challenged by evidence that synaptic use may result in inhibition rather than facilitation. Bliss et al.,[11] following conditioning experiments in isolated cortical slabs, concluded that the great majority of pathways examined must have contained synaptic functions that were less likely to transmit excitation the more often the pathway was used. Creutzfeldt[22] concluded that intracortical inhibition plays an essential, if not the exclusive, role for the elaboration of the peculiar response properties and "trigger features" of cortical neurons. His findings indicate that over a distance of 300–400 m each cortical neuron is inhibited by its neighbors and that the individual cortical connections (he emphasizes the existence of a large number of intracortical fibers) are essentially and dominantly inhibitory. The cortical neurons are not isolated, but rather are included in a network of intracortical connections; the cortical module is a cylinder of 500–1,000 m, and neurons in the center would be inhibited by other neurons in the cylinder. The cylinder is not a column; it is repeated continuously, and each neuron is again the center of such a cylinder. It represents the organization of a network, rather than a mosaic.[22] He notes that Phillips[59] has described a comparable network for the motor system. Throughout his analysis, Creutzfeldt emphasized the parallel rather than the hierarchical processing of information.

Unmasking, which has been discussed in detail elsewhere,[4, 5, 30, 70] may relate to the balance of excitation and inhibition. Wall's[70] studies of sensory inputs to the spinal cord demonstrate how sensory loss can reveal neural connections that are heavily inhibited in the normal state. He suggests that this process may use diverse connections that have been laid down in the embryo but had been previously inhibited during maturation.

Modification of Reflexes.—Until recently, reflexes, especially the primitive reflexes, were considered rather immutable. However, it is now known that even primitive reflexes such as the vestibular ocular response can be modified and even reversed with training.[49] Tendon transfer often requires this to be so; in 1941 Weiss and Brown[73] first showed reflex modification to be possible with transfer of the biceps femoris tendon to replace a paralyzed quadricep in children with polio. Thus, the flexor muscle had to become incorporated into extensor patterns. While this was easily accomplished, a reversion to its flexor role could occur even a long time following surgery if the patient was fatigued.

Modification of the reflexes is, of course, a natural phenomenon. The normal Babinski reflex of an infant becomes suppressed during development, but a brain lesion can unmask the suppressed reflex.

NEUROTRANSMITTERS

One of the exciting new areas of stroke rehabilitation research is the role of specific neurotransmitters in functional recovery. Their findings have emerged from the demonstration of the presence of large numbers of neuroactive substances, some of which are concentrated in specific parts of the brain. Much of the following is taken from a section prepared by one of us (P.B.) for the American Academy of Physical Medicine and Rehabilitation syllabus chapter entitled "Rehabilitation in Brain Disorders."[1]

In the past, the cellular organization of the brain has been studied by classic histological and silver impregnation techniques. It is now possible to map chemically defined neuronal systems, which do not necessarily correspond to those described by the morphological techniques. The chemical categorization, largely by classes of neurotransmitters, is leading to a greatly increased understanding of normal function, of the causes of some diseases, and of drug action mechanisms. In addition, some studies[60] are providing evidence on the effects of specific training on neurotransmitters, and thus on the relationship of neurotransmitters to brain plasticity. Approximately three dozen substances fulfill the criteria for neurotransmitters, and more are being discovered. In addition, there is strong evidence that a number of other naturally occurring substances, including the neuroactive peptides, amino acids, and cyclic nucleotides, also function as neurotransmitters or as modulators of neural function.

Certain substances have more or less invariable actions: gamma aminobutyric acid and glycine inhibit, while glutamate and aspartate excite. Others have differing effects depending upon the nature of the cell in which receptors are being tested. Thus acetylcholine frequently excites, but can also inhibit, whereas dopamine, norepinephrine, and serotonin almost always inhibit, but have some excitatory actions. Most of the neuroactive substances are secreted at synapses; they are generally found in the highest concentrations in the presynaptic terminals except for neurohormones and some neuromodulators. It is generally accepted (in spite of some contrary evidence) that transmitter molecules are stored within vesicles in the nerve terminal and that a calcium-dependent excitation-secretion coupling within the nerve terminal requires the transient exchange of vesicular contents into the synaptic cleft. The receptors for all of the neurotransmitters studied to date are localized on the surface of the cell. Only those receptors for steroid and thyroid hormones are apparently intracellular.[21]

Among the most interesting neurotransmitters are the catecholamines, in particular dopamine and its metabolic products in the mammalian brain, norepinephrine and epinephrine. Dopamine, which comprises more than 50% of the CNS catecholamines, has a widely different distribution than epinephrine, and thus is not only its precursor. In parkinsonism, there are degenerative changes in the substantia nigra and partial destruction of dopamine neurons. Knowledge of the effects of disease processes on specific transmitter systems has led to effective use of L-dopa therapy for parkinsonism. Another important catecholamine mechanism in the CNS is mediated by the locus ceruleus in the caudal pons. The fibers from this nucleus form five major noradrenergic tracks, which virtually encompass the brain and cerebellum. A major effect of activating these pathways is the inhibition of spontaneous discharges, resulting in a slow type of synaptic transaction in which the hyperpolarizing response of the target cells is accompanied by increased membrane resistance.[21] Since the fibers from this small nucleus are so widespread (for example, from the locus ceruleus they sweep around the frontal pole of the brain before coursing across the top of the brain), many injuries to the brain produce some destruction of locus ceruleus fibers. One consequence of the damage to a terminal field projection site of the locus ceruleus is that a depression in locus ceruleus functioning occurs that affects areas remote from the primary injury site.[12] That is perhaps, for repair purposes, related to a shift in the locus ceruleus from neurotransmitter production to protein synthesis.[63] The depression in locus ceruleus functioning may be largely responsible for the transient behavioral dysfunctions observed after cortical injuries, since either amphetamine (but not apomorphine) or intraventricularly administered norepinephrine (but not dopamine) permanently accelerates recovery of function when a single dose is given shortly after injury[12, 28] (unpublished observations). Drugs that block norepinephrine functioning also retard recovery of function.[12, 28, 29] It is particularly interesting to note that neither the retarded nor the accelerated recovery occurs in the absence of a concomitant rehabilitation program.[28]

Although the recovery of function from the transient symptoms is normally permanent, the brain is still in a vulnerable state. For example, it is possible to reinstate unilateral sensorimotor deficits in recovered animals by administration of phenoxybenzamine (an alpha-adrenergic antagonist) but not by propranolol (a beta-adrenergic antagonist) or haloperidol.[12, 29] These results indicate that not only is norepinephrine involved in maintaining the observed recovery, but that certain drugs may be contraindicated following brain injuries.

The recent studies on catecholamines and other neuroactive substances suggest an exciting future for neuropharmacological therapies for stroke in combination with appropriate physical and other therapies.

THE ROLE OF ENVIRONMENTS IN RECOVERY OF FUNCTION

Human and animal studies have revealed that the environment has an influence on recovery. For example, a large number that could be classed as rehabilitation studies have been undertaken with rats. The principal rehabilitation procedure has been manipulation of the environment.[72] These studies began with a pioneering experiment completed by Schwartz[64] demonstrating that allowing rats to experience an enriched environment for 3 months after occipital cortex lesions significantly improved their maze test scores.

Rosenzweig and collaborators (summarized in Rosenzweig[60]) were able to induce significant changes in brain anatomy and brain chemistry in young as well as adult nonlesioned rats by giving them differential experience in one of three environments: standard colony cages (SC), a more enriched condition (EC) (which can be considered to be comparable to a rehabilitation program), or isolated in an impoverished condition (IC). The EC rats developed significantly greater cortical measures (tissue weight, total acetylcholinesterase activity, total cholinesterase, and cortical depth) than their restricted environment littermates. Most of these measures were significantly greater in the occipital region of the cortex than in other cortical areas. Furthermore, these EC effects on occipital cortical measures were also noted in rats blinded at birth.[61, 62] The neuroanatomical effects of environmental complexity have been reviewed by Walsh.[71] Although the EC in most experiments was available 24 hours per day, a period of 2 hours per day was found to be as effective as 24 hours.[61]

The results with maze tests provide strong evidence that enriched experience promotes overall recovery of function: good scores on the series of maze tests require a combination of sensorimotor capacities, motivation, learning, and memory. Unfortunately a deficit in any one of these capacities results in inferior performance. Optimal recovery, at least for the rat, is not obtained simply by restoration of general health, and certainly not by protecting the individual from stimulation as in the IC environment, nor simply by providing socialization, but rather by providing complex stimulation and opportunities for experience.[60]

Although stroke patients are not kept in environments comparable to the IC rats in these experiments, a patient receiving intravenous medication is kept relatively immobile to avoid displacing the needle, and is, in addition to the motor restriction, in a sensory deprived environment in a hospital room. Being placed in an intensive care unit compounds the environmental deficits: many, if not most, patients in intensive care units have some periods of psychological disorientation.[56] Improving the environment in such units may reduce the incidence of such psychiatric complications[37]; for example, over twice as many episodes of organic delirium were seen in the intensive care unit without windows, in comparison to a unit with windows.[74] The effects of these environmental factors on the mortality and morbidity of patients has yet to be determined. In the postacute phase, patients kept in a rehabilitation ward are in unfamiliar, often hostile environments, deprived of family and home. Often, rehabilitation facilities are located in the basement or in other harsh settings. These and other environmental factors may influence rehabilitation outcome. In fact, recent evidence has shown that the view through the window may influence recovery from surgery: Ulrich[69] showed that surgical patients assigned to rooms with windows looking out on a natural scene had shorter postoperative hospital stays, received fewer negative evaluative comments in nurse's notes, and took fewer potent analgesics than matched patients in similar rooms with windows facing a brick building wall.

The appropriate environment for therapy is a subject of clinical importance. Whereas group activities and peer interactions may be appropriate for certain groups of patients, other patients, and in particular certain therapeutic interventions, require complete concentration and a quiet environment. For example, electromyographic sensory feedback for developing neuromuscular control ideally requires quiet individual rooms due to the high level of concentration required (see signal-to-noise ratio discussion below).

The therapeutic environment also includes the home and social environments. This has been well recognized and has been incorporated into most long-term inpatient rehabilitation programs by means of the judicious use of home leaves and weekend passes. In fact, a supportive family member may be able to undertake rehabilitation interventions that, although less technically developed than professional therapy, may be able to achieve significant functional gains in the familiar and supportive environment of the home; specific therapeutic activities may be more closely related to the patient's particular interests (see case discussed by Bach-y-Rita,[3] pp. 240–243). Research into the effects of the various therapy environments may lead to the most appropriate use, at different stages of evolution of the stroke patient, of acute hospital bedside rehabilitation, rehabilitation units in acute hospitals, late (chronic) rehabilitation units, specific rehabilitation hospitals, community rehabilitation facilities, nursing homes, and home programs.

THE POSTACUTE REHABILITATION PROGRAM

LEARNING AND RECOVERY

The problem of retraining the postacute patient often is one of information processing rather than a lack of inherent ability or spontaneous recovery. There is no reason to believe that with proper training the learning process associated with neuromuscular reeducation cannot be a continuation of normal adaptive motor programming. In the case of stroke and its resultant brain injury, motor control may be dysfunctional or functional. The patient may or may not be aware if his motor programs are inappropriate or even if his sensory mechanisms (i.e., proprioceptive and kinesthetic sensibility) are dysfunctional. The rehabilitation potential of any patient (acute or postacute) depends not only upon the level of the lesion(s), but also on the reestablishment of information inputs to the sensory association areas of the brain that direct or redirect motor programming.

Although the overall sequence of neuronal mechanisms involved in neuromuscular retraining is not well understood, it is currently thought (as reviewed by Wolf[75]) that information concerning a volitional movement is processed by the cortical sensorimotor and association areas in conjunction with the lateral cerebellum, basal ganglia, and the premotor cortex. The basal ganglia and cerebellum, which have multiple inputs from many locations in the brain, may inhibit or excite this activity depending upon information received from the thalamus and the somatosensory, visual, and auditory cortices. The cerebellum also contains motor sequence programs that allow preprogrammed, and particularly relatively fast, movements to occur.

Volitional motor control programs are modified and memorized primarily through associative learning. For this sequence to occur purposely and correctly, millions of neurons from many areas in the brain must be reprogrammed and allowed to operate under the most ideal conditions that can be made available. We agree with Josephine Moore[53] when she comments on this situation:

Each successive synapse [is modified] by the circumstances of the moment, the immediate future, and the past, or the organism's genetic heritage coupled with learned and/or environmental experiences that have been incorporated into its nervous system.

SENSORY FEEDBACK THERAPY

In the forefront of research concerning the postacute neuromuscular retraining of neuromuscular dysfunction has been the use of EMG sensory (bio)feedback therapy. Studies using EMG feedback have been conducted in the retraining of postacute stroke and brain injury.[2, 9, 15, 16, 31, 33, 36, 40, 41, 43, 44, 47, 50, 55, 66, 76, 77] All of these studies have used similar methods, with many demonstrating significant upper- and lower-extremity functional return in patients who had been functionally disabled for 5 or more years. The largest of these studies was reported in 1979 by Brudny et al.[16] They reported on 150 postacute neuromuscular disability patients. Using the visual and auditory feedback from surface-electrode EMG, they were able to successfully habituate synergy patterns, facilitate muscle control in seemingly paralyzed muscles, and reestablish certain functional abilities in more than half of these patients.

In our clinic the use of EMG sensory feedback in the neuromuscular retraining of stroke patients typically consists of five interactive steps.[8] The first involves (1) general relaxation, including the uninvolved extremity. Once this low-noise baseline (see below) is established, (2) slow, reciprocal motor control of the uninvolved extremity is acquired. (3) This relatively slow motor control paradigm is used as a model to suppress unnecessary muscle activity and/or to facilitate voluntary contractions of the involved extremity. (4) Voluntary reciprocal sequencing of the involved side is then partially established and (5) is used to generalize appropriate proprioceptive and kinesthetic sensibility of the individual muscles and joints to functional tasks requiring more integrative motor control sequences. Repetitions of this sequence in the clinic, as well as simple (usually non-EMG) exercises at home, usually allow the patient to regain some amount of function.

Electromyographic feedback should be considered as one of many therapy methods that can provide "sensory feedback" required for neuromuscular retraining. Effective neuromuscular retraining does not depend upon the exact device that may be utilized, but rather on the overall information transmittal characteristics that are associated with the particular therapy strategy. Clearly, the therapist must not only know how to use the EMG; the therapist must also know how to apply manual facilitation techniques such as quick stretching (reflex), palpatation, and patterning to promote EMG responses. The EMG works best in the hands of the therapist who knows many modalities. The EMG simply acts as a sensory facilitator or substitution device, thus increasing the patient's and the therapist's proprioceptive inputs, both in quantity and quality, until the patient can reacquire motor control that can be normally sensed without the EMG. However, it is the therapist that must actually help the patient initiate the correct motor commands and inhibit the incorrect motor commands through modalities that normally might have been insufficient to produce any apparent response. Accordingly, a very experienced therapist may often not require such a "high-tech" device, if she/he can provide sufficient sensory feedback information concerning the patient's ongoing neuromuscular status with some other method of facilitation, i.e., active assist, range of motion, mirror exercises, etc.

Ultimately a combination of many factors determines success or failure with a patient. The control of these factors is particularly important in the postacute patient, because often, in a certain period of time, the patient's motor status becomes stable, and thus spontaneous recovery is of little or no help; the establishment of optimal (re)training conditions are imperative.

THE CONCEPT OF SIGNAL-TO-NOISE RATIO (S/N) IN REHABILITATION[8]

In neuromuscular rehabilitation, sensory feedback information not only includes information processed by an EMG; it includes any cortically processed afferent input. Neural adaptation or plasticity in this case does not include regeneration, but rather, as previously mentioned, probably the unmasking of parallel pathways or the resolution of diaschisis through differential activation of CNS synapses.[4, 5, 30, 70] The basic concept of dividing a signal by it associated noise to obtain a ratio S/N should be considered when examining the optimization of any therapy procedure or learning paradigm. Traditionally, S/N has been a term used in electrical engineering to give estimates of dynamic range of an electrical device. It is a relative measure of the device's effectiveness in increasing wanted characteristics (signal) while decreasing unwanted characteristics (noise). For example, as expressed with the logarithmic dB scale, an old Edison record has a maximum S/N of 30 dB, while a laser disc is thousands of times more effective with a S/N of about 95 dB. The increased information capacity of the laser disc is a result of not only its ability to provide a wide frequency response (signal), but also by what signals it does not transmit (noise). The virtual perfection of the laser disc would not be possible without its low noise properties.

Similarly, since the 1920s, the effectiveness of amplification systems for listeners with sensorineural hearing impairment has been quantitatively described with respect to hearing loss and speech intelligibility with relatively simple signal/noise relationships. One such relationship has been represented by the following articulation index (A) equation:[58]

$$A = P\int_0^\infty I(F)W(F)df.$$

I(F) indicates the importance of different frequencies to speech intelligibility. W(F) is slightly less than or equal to unity and indicates the amount of available information delivered to the listener under less than optimal conditions. P is a proficiency factor that measures how precise the talker's enunciation of the speech material is as well as how experienced the listener is in listening to the talker.

The complete understanding of this equation is not possible in this chapter. The concept of such an equation is significant to neuromuscular rehabilitation because it demonstrates that the net effectiveness of two people transmitting and receiving information through differing devices and environmental conditions can be evaluated. This is similar to when a therapist communicates with a patient. It may be possible to consider the effectiveness of any neuromuscular rehabilitation procedure with some form of S/N relation. Unfortunately, it is currently impossible to quantify the effectiveness of neuromuscular therapy. Nevertheless, for discussion purposes, it is possible to predict certain qualitative S/N factors that could affect patient rehabilitation. The following factors are not disassociated from the patient's neurologic lesion; they are primarily concerned with environmental factors and are not meant to be exhaustive.

Patient and Therapist Participation.—It can be theorized that active patient involvement probably increases the S/N by both allowing the patient the opportunity to better attend to retraining information (signal) while disregarding other information that is not related to actual retraining and proper functional motor control (noise). This is reinforced by animal and human research indicating that learning is a conscious and cortically organized process.[30] Therefore, passive "participation" relative to learning may in fact be impossible. This does not mean that passive treatment techniques should not be used to promote range of motion and decrease the risk of contractures. In addition, automatic and functional movement patterns should be utilized to promote proprioception and kinesthetic sensibility as to provide cortical afference and facilitate "active" participation that is required for retraining to take place.

Ultimately, it is the patient who really trains the patient. The therapist is a guide; his/her modalities act as a source of information and therefore of feedback. For this reason, the most effective strategy is to train the patient to be his/her own best therapist as soon as possible. This can be maximized with the help of friends and family who can be trained to perform simple facilitation, to give verbal reminders as to correct behaviors, to help keep track of progress on goal attainment sheets, and/or to simply provide positive moral support. Similarly, the patient can also be taught basic anatomy, physiology, and kinesiology as related to their condition in order to decrease their dependency on the rehabilitation professional as the expert who will do something to cure him. This provides added information (signal), but it also helps increase receptivity (decrease noise).

Relatively large amounts of patient-conducted home training provide a substantial amount of cost-free therapy, thus extending therapy resources over a larger period of time and to more patients. Programs consisting of patient education and at least a 20:1 ratio of home-to-clinic training have been demonstrated to be successful in differing postacute retraining situations.[9, 10] Even with optimal modalities, successful treatment cannot occur without a positive attitude and resulting encouragement from the therapist. This should include a positive involvement in not only the patient's physical condition, but also their psychosocial condition. The effectiveness of information transfer and its assimilation is critically dependent upon the reduction of such noise components. In two therapy situations (assuming $E = S/N$) that have the same incoming signal strength or method ($S_1 = S_2$), with all other variables also equal, the situation that has the lowest noise (if $N_1 < N_2$) must always have the greatest effectiveness (therefore, $E_1 > E_2$). Particularly in the postacute patient, covert psychosocial issues may appear as a physiologic plateau. These problems can act as shields that are impenetrable to even the most effective therapy modalities.

It is easily understood that under conditions of equivalent noise ($N_1 = N_2$), the therapy situation with the most effective signal or best method (if $S_1 > S_2$) will always have the greatest effectiveness (therefore, $E_1 > E_2$). Similarly, various techniques can be used to increase (signal) strength. For example, any modality can be augmented with videotape or Polaroid film feedback.[10] This provides long-term feedback to both the patient and the therapist. This long-term feedback signal helps provide information regarding specific or gross changes in function that can occur so slowly in the postacute patient. Also, the use of inexpensive goal-attainment graphs can help supply short-term feedback in the EMG upper-extremity neuromuscular retraining of chronic stroke patients with impaired expressive and auditory comprehension.[8]

Efficiency of Modality as Related to Environment.—Most therapy is conducted in a "gym" environment where many patients are being treated by many therapists. This certainly provides strong socialization inputs to both patient and therapist. However, most therapists will agree that this is not an ideal environment for the acute stroke patient, who is disoriented and can be seen to respond to "everything in the room." What about the postacute stroke patient who demonstrates no cognitive deficits? Typically, this type of patient would be trained with many other patients and therapists in close proximity.

Home treatment might even include exercises that could be conveniently done in front of the television. However, noisy conditions might be satisfactory for developing muscle strength or maintaining passive range of motion, but they are not optimal for the development of neuromuscular programs. A child does not learn to play the piano near an orchestra. Instead, he learns in isolation, where he can have optimal conditions to concentrate, i.e., receive positive and negative feedback and repeatedly modify his neuromuscular programs that will eventually allow him to play the piano successfully. It would be advantageous for the child to occasionally meet others who were practicing, particularly at differing stages of development, but he typically would not "practice" with them. Similarly, a patient who is trying to reestablish neuromuscular control should be involved in support groups, but should "practice" in a quiet individual room where concentration can be maximized.

Nonrepetitious Repetitions.—Active patient awareness is essential to the information processing and the reprogramming of motor control. It is therefore important that repetitions be performed in a manner that does not involve tedious repetition. New neuromuscular programs cannot be reinforced if previous programs are reinforced. Old programs such as compensatory or dyscoordinated movements are perpetuated when the patient is allowed to move relatively fast or imprecisely. Uninteresting and/or nonfunctional tasks will eventuate in fast, imprecise, and improper motor control. As Kottke has explained,[46]

A person cannot monitor a control activity to cause isolated contraction of a prime mover and maintain relaxation of all other muscles unless the activity is slow. If the activity is rapid . . . the increased effort causes irradiation of impulses transcerebrally and through internuncial synapses to produce cocontractions of other muscles. Coordination develops only as a result of prolonged precise practice of elementary units of each pattern of activity.

If unchecked, improper motor control can become a highly reinforced program (see below). Instead, patients must correctly repeat desired motor programs in a manner that maintains alertness and motivation, such as by the use of finely spaced goal attainment and by varying the therapy modalities. These volitional motor control sequences will ultimately have to be practiced thousands of times in order to eventually store a new motor program that is relatively fast, i.e., automatic, coordinated, effortless, functional, and generalizable.

Optimal and Contraindicated Retraining as Related to Possible Abnormal Muscle Recruitment.—For two decades it has been known that there is usually an orderly and additive recruitment in the size of motoneurons and their corresponding muscle fibers in normal animals and man. These motor units seem to be recruited in order from a low- to high-voltage threshold, thus causing an increase in strength of voluntary muscle contraction. The smaller, slower, and weaker motor units are recruited before the larger, faster, and stronger motor units.[38, 39] This orderly recruitment has also been demonstrated for both slow steady movements and for fast ballistic movements in limbs as well as eye muscles[78]; typically, larger units are evident at a relatively high recruitment threshold in a slow ramp contraction, but are not selectively recruited under rapid movement conditions (for review, see Desmedt[25]).

There have been some reported exceptions to this rule.[18–20, 23, 24, 26, 27, 35, 45, 65] One example of deordering in normal humans has been in a multifunctional muscle (first dorsal interosseous) when it was used as a synergist with the thumb in a functional pinch rather than as a prime mover (reviewed by Desmedt[25]). In this situation, the actual contact and even small-pinch combination facilitated primarily higher-threshold (large) motor units; lower-threshold (small) motor units were typically not involved. This neurologic strategy apparently helps ensure a substantial grip that will not be as susceptible to slippage at relatively low-touch prehension thresholds. It is not known how many other special neuronal programs may exist relative to functional tasks.

Because most neuromuscular disorders cause muscle weakness and decreased active range of motion, it is of interest to investigate CNS motor unit recruitment in various neurologic patients. Recent work has found that normal recruitment occurs during simple, nonfunctional isometric contractions in patients with motoneuron disease such as amyotrophic lateral sclerosis and pressure or entrapment neuropathies. However, patients with neurologic disorders such as complete nerve transection with surgical reunion, postacute polymyositis (muscle fiber disease),[52] and parkinsonism[51] demonstrate substantial disorders in recruitment. It appears that when muscle tension feedback is diminished or when correspondence between central and peripheral components of the motoneurons is substantially changed, muscle recruitment becomes disordered, resulting in neuromuscular dysfunction. This disordering will even occur when the number of motor units is within normal limits (reviewed by Milner-Brown et al.[52]). Work remains to be done in the majority of neurologic patients (i.e., brain and spinal cord injury) to determine their muscle recruitment patterns.

Nevertheless, with the above studies in mind, it seems judicious to require that certain patients, such as a stroke patient who has sensory deficits and/or severe flexion synergy, perform their neuromuscular retraining in a manner that perpetuates slow (tonic) muscle control associated with low-threshold motor units. Therapeutic exercises that involve relatively fast repetitions or heavy weights may not do more than promote relatively fast (phasic) muscle control associated with high-threshold motor units, resulting in relatively uncontrolled and rapidly fatiguable motor control, instead of fine and fast fatigue-resistant motor control. Relatively fast movements should probably only be utilized during the final end points of therapy that include more developed and skilled functional activities. This problem might occur in any patient who had a predisposition to disordering and was trying to (re)learn precise motor control or when such control was used as a coactivator in the maintenance of constant or graded movements.

The "Science" of Neuromuscular Recovery.—Fortunately, in just the last few years, there have been rapidly evolving advances in computer science, digital electronics, and applied mathematics that have resulted in the availability of brain imaging techniques that can either provide or have the theoretical potential to provide morphological and functional anatomical images of the brain. Specifically, the combination of computerized tomography, nuclear magnetic resonance (NMR), and positron emission tomography now present previously unavailable opportunities to study the structure and function of the living brain. We are now in our infancy regarding a full understanding of the potential innovative applications of these techniques to stroke recovery.

These new tools are of particular value because, although recovery of function has been previously demonstrated in both animal and clinical studies, clinical rehabilitation procedures for brain-damaged patients have, to a large extent, evolved in the absence of solid physiologic research data. We still do not know how, where, or why recovery takes place after stroke. This information is essential to the development of efficient rehabilitation programs and to the optimization of human potential in the injured brain. The answers to these questions can no longer be provided by single individuals or disciplines. Interdisciplinary efforts are necessary to investigate the potential of these new capabilities as applied to the theory of CNS recovery and to the improvement of clinical rehabilitation strategies.

In summary, it is apparent that we have the ability today to increase function in many patients. Regardless of the methods involved in retraining, the following principles seem basic to motor control and its reacquisition:

1. Optimal existing motor control depends upon optimal sensory feedback information or measures.
2. Optimal neural adaptation or plasticity of motor control reprogramming depends upon the optimization of sensory information.

3. Optimal utilization of sensory feedback information depends upon (the establishment of) conditions that provide the highest possible S/N of that information.

The components of optimal sensory feedback information must extend far beyond the availability of technology, such as therapeutic EMG. If carefully performed, therapeutic exercise should similarly provide high amounts of proprioceptive and kinesthetic feedback. In addition, it is important to remember that environment can substantially decrease the patient's ability to process available sensory feedback information, thus reducing his net rehabilitation potential. This not only includes crowded and/or noisy therapy conditions, but also psychosocial factors involving the patient at home and/or his interactions with the therapist. On the other hand, the patient's rehabilitation potential also depends on the creativity, imagination, and persistence of the therapy staff. Any one of these factors can limit or halt patient progress.

REFERENCES

1. *Syllabus Chapter: Rehabilitation in Brain Disorders.* Chicago, American Academy of Physical Medicine and Rehabilitation, 1985.
2. Andrews JM: Neuromuscular re-education of the hemiplegic with the aid of the electromyograph. *Arch Phys Med Rehabil* 1964; 45:530–532.
3. Bach-y-Rita P (ed): *Recovery of Function: Theoretical Considerations for Brain Injury Rehabilitation.* Baltimore, University Park Press, 1980.
4. Bach-y-Rita P: Central nervous system lesions: Sprouting and unmasking in rehabilitation. *Arch Phys Med Rehabil* 1981a; 62:413–417.
5. Bach-y-Rita P: Brain plasticity as a basis for the development of rehabilitation procedures for hemiplegia. *Scand J Rehabil Med* 1981b; 13:73–83.
6. Bach-y-Rita P (ed): Rehabilitation following brain damage: Some neurophysiological mechanisms. *Int Rehabil Med* 1982; 4:165–199.

7. Bach-y-Rita P: The process of recovery from stroke, in Brandstater ME (ed): *Stroke Rehabilitation.* Baltimore, Williams & Wilkins Co, (in press).

8. Balliet R: Motor control strategies in the retraining of facial paralysis, in *Proceedings of the Vth International Symposium on the Facial Nerve.* Paris, Masson, SA, 1985.

9. Balliet R, Levy B, Blood KMT: Upper extremity sensory feedback therapy (SFT) in chronic patients with impaired expressive and auditory comprehension. *Arch Phys Med Rehabil* 1986; 67:304–310.

10. Balliet R, Shinn JB, Bach-y-Rita P: Facial paralysis rehabilitation: Retraining selective muscle control. *Int Rehabil Med* 1982; 4:67–74.

11. Bliss, TVP, Burns BD, Uttley AM: Factors affecting the conductivity of pathways in the cerebral cortex. *J Physiol* 1968; 195:339–367.

12. Boyeson MG, Feeney DM: The role of norepinephrine in recovery from brain injury. *Neurosci Abstr* 1984; 10:68.

13. Brinkman J, Kuypers HGJM: Cerebral control of contralateral and ipsilateral arm, hand and finger movements in the split-brain Rhesus monkey. *Brain* 1973; 96:653–674.

14. Brodal A: Self-observations and neuroanatomical considerations after a stroke. *Brain* 1973; 96:675–694.

15. Brudny J, Korein J, Grynbaum BB, et al: EMG feedback therapy: Review of treatment of 114 patients. *Arch Phys Med Rehabil* 1976; 57:55–61.

16. Brudny J, Korein J, Grynbaum BB, et al: Helping hemiparetics to help themselves. *JAMA* 1979; 241:814–818.

17. Brunnstrom S: *Movement Therapy in Hemiplegia.* New York, Harper & Row, 1970.

18. Burke RE: Group Ia synaptic input to fast and slow twitch motor units of cat tricep surae. *J Physiol* 1968; 196:605–630.

19. Burke RE: Motor unit recruitment: What are the critical factors? in Desmedt JE (ed): *Motor Unit Types Recruitment and Plasticity in Health and Disease: Progress in Clinical Neurophysiology.* Basel, Karger, 1981; pp 61–84.

20. Burke RE, Edgerton VR: Motor unit properties and selective involvement in movement. *Exerc Sport Sci Rev* 1975; 3:31–69.

21. Cooper JR, Bloom FE, Roth RH: *The Biochemical Basis of Neu-*

ropharmacology, ed 4. New York, Oxford University Press, 1982.

22. Creutzfeldt O: Some problems of cortical organization in the light of ideas of the classical "Hirnpathologie" and of modern neurophysiology, in Zulch KJ, Creutzfeldt O, Galbraith GC (eds): *Cerebral Localization.* Berlin, Springer, 1975, pp 217–226.

23. Desmedt JE: Patterns of motor commands during various types of voluntary movement in man. *Trends Neurosci* 1980; 3:265–268.

24. Desmedt JE: Plasticity of motor unit organization studies by coherent electromyography in patients with nerve lesions or with myopathic or neuropathic diseases, in Desmedt JE (ed): *Motor Unit Types, Recruitment and Plasticity in Health and Disease: Progress in Clinical Neurophysiology.* Karger, 1981; pp 250–304.

25. Desmedt JE: Size principle of motoneuron recruitment and the calibration of muscle force and speed in man, in Desmedt JE (ed): *Motor Control Mechanisms in Health and Disease.* New York, Raven Press 1983; 227–251.

26. Desmedt JE, Godaux E: Spinal motoneuron recruitment in man: Deordering with direction, but not with speed of voluntary movement. *Science* 1981; 214:933–936.

27. Edgerton VR, Cremer S: Motor unit plasticity and possible mechanisms, in Desmedt JE (ed): *Motor Unit Types, Recruitment and Plasticity in Health and Disease: Progress in Clinical Neurophysiology.* Basel, Karger, 1981, pp 220–240.

28. Feeney DM, Gonzalez A, Law WA: Amphetamine haloperidol and experience interact to affect rate of recovery after motor cortex lesion. *Science* 1982; 217:855–857.

29. Feeney D, Hovda DA, Salo A: Phenoxybenzamine reinstates all motor and sensory deficits in cats fully recovered from sensorimotor cortex ablations. *FASEB* 1983; 42:1157.

30. Finger S, Stein DG: *Brain Damage and Recovery.* New York, Academic Press, 1982.

31. Flom RP, Quast JE, Boller JD, et al: Biofeedback training to overcome post stroke foot-drop. *Geriatrics* 1976; 31:47–51.

32. Gardner WJ: Removal of the right cerebral hemisphere for infiltrating glioma. *JAMA* 1933; 101:823–826.

33. Gianutos JG, Eberstein A, Krasilovsky G, et al: EMG feedback in

the rehabilitation of upper extremity function: Single case studies of chronic hemiplegics. *International Neuropsychological Society Bulletin: Symposium Issue* 1979, p 12.

34. Glees P: Functional reorganization following hemispherectomy in man and after small experimental lesions in primates, in Bach-y-Rita P, (ed): *Recovery of Function: Theoretical Considerations for Brain Injury Rehabilitation.* Baltimore, University Park Press, 1980, pp 106–126.

35. Grimby L, Hannerz J: Flexibility of recruitment order of continuously and intermittently discharging motor units in voluntary contraction, in Desmedt JE (ed): *Motor Unit Types, Recruitment and Plasticity in Health and Disease: Progress in Clinical Neurophysiology.* Basel, Karger, 1981, vol 9, pp 201–221.

36. Harris JD: The value of electromyograph-monitored muscle re-education of the hemiplegic arm. *Osteopath Assoc* 1970; 10:222–232.

37. Heller SS, Franke KA, Malm JR, et al: Psychiatric complications of open heart surgery. *N Engl J Med* 1970; 283:1015–1019.

38. Henneman E, Somjen G, Carpenter DD: Functional significance of cell size in spinal motoneurons. *J Neurophysiol* 1965a; 28:560–580.

39. Henneman E, Somjen G, Carpenter DO: Excitability and inhibility of motoneurons of different sizes. *J Neurophysiol* 1965b; 28:599–620.

40. Hurd W, Pegram V, Nepomuceno C: Comparison of actual and simulated EMG biofeedback in the treatment of hemiplegic patients. *Am J Phys Med* 1980; 59:73–82.

41. Inglis J, Donald MW, Monga TN, et al: Electromyographic biofeedback and physical therapy of the hemiplegic upper limb. *Arch Phys Med Rehabil* 1984; 65:755–759.

42. Jebson RH, Griffith ER, Long EW, et al: Function of "normal" hand in stroke patients. *Arch Phys Med Rehabil* 1971; 51:170–181.

43. Johnson HE, Garton WH: Muscle re-education in hemiplegia by use of electromyographic device. *Arch Phys Med Rehabil* 1973; 54:320–323.

44. Kelly J, Belver M, Wolf S: Procedures for EMG biofeedback training in medical upper extremities of hemiplegic patients. *Phys Ther* 1979; 59:1500–1507.

45. Kernell D: Functional properties of spinal motoneurons and gra-

dation of muscle force, in Desmedt JE (ed): *Motor Control Mechanisms in Health and Disease.* New York, Raven Press, 1983, pp 213–226.

46. Kottke F: The neurophysiology of motor function, in Kottke F, Stillwell GK, Lehmann JF (eds): *Krusen's Handbook of Physical Medicine and Rehabilitation.* Philadelphia, WB Saunders Co, 1982, pp 218–253.

47. Lee K, Hill E, Johnston R, et al: Myofeedback for muscle retraining in hemiplegia patients. *Arch Phys Med Rehabil* 1976; 57:588–591.

48. McClanahan M, Vigano S: *Evaluation of Sensory Motor Function of the "Uninvolved" Upper Extremity of Patients with Unilateral Brain Damage from Stroke,* thesis. Division of Physical Therapy, Stanford University, Stanford, Calif 1978.

49. Melvill Jones G, Gonshor A: Goal-directed flexibility in the vestibulo-ocular reflex arc, in Lennerstrand G, Bach-y-Rita P (eds): *Basic Mechanisms of Ocular Motility and Their Clinical Implications.* Oxford, Pergamon Press, 1975, pp 227–245.

50. Middaugh SJ, Miller MC: Electromyographic feedback; effect on voluntary contractions in paretic subjects. *Arch Phys Med Rehabil* 1980; 61:24–29.

51. Milner-Brown HS, Fisher MA, Weiner WJ: Electrical properties of motor units in Parkinsonism and a possible relationship with bradykinesia. *J Neurol Neurosurg Psychiatry* 1979; 42:35–41.

52. Milner-Brown HS, Stein RB, Lee RG et al: Motor unit recruitment in patients with neuromuscular disorders, in Desmedt JE (ed): *Motor Unit Types, Recruitment and Plasticity in Health and Disease: Progress in Clincial Neurophysiology.* Basel, Karger, 1981, pp 305–318.

53. Moore J: Neuroanatomical considerations relating to recovery of function following brain injury, in Bach-y-Rita P (ed): *Recovery of Function: Theoretical Considerations for Brain Injury Rehabilitation.* Baltimore, University Park Press, 1980, pp 9–90.

54. Mountcastle VB, Lynch JC, Georgopoulos A, et al: Posterior parietal association cortex of monkey: Command functions for operations within extrapersonal space. *J Neurophysiol* 1975; 38:871–908.

55. Mrocyek N, Halpern D, McHugh R: Electromyographic feedback and physical therapy for neuromuscular retraining in hemiplegia. *Arch Phys Med Rehabil* 1978; 59:258–267.

56. Nadelson T: Psychiatric aspects of the intensive care of critically ill patients, in Skillman J (ed): *Intensive Care.* Baltimore, Little, Brown & Co, 1975, pp 36–60.

57. Paillard J: The patterning of skilled movements, in *Handbook of Physiology,* Baltimore, Williams & Wilkins, 1960, vol 3, pp 1679–1708.

58. Pavlovic CV, Studebaker GA: An evaluation of some assumptions underlying the articulation index. *J Acoust Soc Am* 1984; 75(5).

59. Phillips CG: Cortical localization and sensori-motor processes at the "middle level" of primates. *Proc R Soc Med* 1973; 66:987–1002.

60. Rosenzweig M: Animal models for effects of brain lesions and for rehabilitation, in Bach-y-Rita P (ed): *Recovery of Function: Theoretical Considerations for Brain Injury Rehabilitation.* Baltimore, University Park Press, 1980, pp 127–172.

61. Rosenzweig M, Bennett EL, Diamond MC et al: Influences of environmental complexity and visual stimulation on development of occipital cortex in rats. *Brain Res* 1969; 14:427–445.

62. Rosenzweig M, Krech D, Bennett EL, et al: Effects of environmental complexity and training on brain chemistry and anatomy; a replication and extension. *J Comp Physiol Psychol* 1962; 55:429–437.

63. Ross RA, Jah PH, Reis DJ: Reversible changes in the accumulation and activities of pyrazine hydroxylase and dopamine beta hydroxylase in neurons of the locus ceruleus during the retrograde reaction period. *Brain Res* 1975; 92:57–72.

64. Schwartz S: Effect of neonatal cortical lesions and early environmental factors on adult rat behavior. *J Comp Physiol Psychol* 1964; 57:72–77.

65. Stein RB, Bertoldi R: The size principle, in Desmedt JE (ed): *Motor Unit Types, Recruitment and Plasticity in Health and Disease: Progress in Clinical Neurophysiology.* Basel, Karger, 1981, vol 9, pp 85–96.

66. Takebe K, Basmajian JV: Gait analysis in stroke patients to assess treatments of foot-drop. *Arch Phys Med Rehabil* 1976; 57:305–310.

67. Travis AM, Woolsey CN: Motor performance of monkeys after bilateral partial and total cerebral decortication. *Am Phys Med* 1956; 35:273–310.

68. Twitchell TE: The restoration of motor function following hemiplegia in man. *Brain* 1951; 74:433–480.
69. Ulrich RS: View through the window may influence recovery from surgery. *Science* 1984; 224:420–421.
70. Wall PD: Mechanisms of plasticity of connection following damage in adult mammalian nervous systems, in Bach-y-Rita P (ed): *Recovery of Function: Theoretical Considerations for Brain Injury Rehabilitation.* Baltimore, University Park Press, 1980, pp 91–105.
71. Walsh, RN: Effects of environmental complexity and deprivation on brain anatomy and histology: A review, *Int J Neurosci* 1981; 12:33–51.
72. Walsh RN, Greenough WT (eds): *Environments as Therapy for Brain Dysfunction.* New York, Plenum Press, 1976.
73. Weiss PA, Brown P: Electromyographic studies on recoordination of leg movements in poliomyelitis patients with transposed tendons. *Proc Soc Exp Biol* 1941; 48:284–287.
74. Wilson LM: Intensive care delirium: The effect of outside deprivation in windowless units. *Arch Intern Med* 1975; 130:225–226.
75. Wolf SE: Neurophysiological factors in electromyographic feedback for neuromotor disturbances, in Basmajian JV (ed): *Biofeedback: Principles and Practice for Clinicians.* Baltimore, Williams & Wilkins Co, 1983, pp 1–22.
76. Wolf SL, Baker MP, Kelly JL: EMG biofeedback in stroke: Effect of patient characteristics. *Arch Phys Med Rehabil* 1979; 60:92–102.
77. Wolf SL, Baker MP, Kelly JL: EMG biofeedback in stroke: A 1-year follow-up on the effect of patient characteristics. *Arch Phys Med Rehabil* 1980; 61:351–355.
78. Yamanaka Y, Bach-y-Rita P: Conduction velocities in the abducens nerve correlated with vestibular mystagmus in cats. *Exp Neurol* 1968; 20:143–155.

4

Motor Learning Considerations in Stroke Rehabilitation

Carolee J. Winstein, M.S., P.T.

Previous literature has described the complex nature of problems involved in the rehabilitation of the stroke victim. Consideration has been given to the neuromuscular, sensory, perceptual, psychological, sociological, and prognostic issues relevant to the physical therapist. However, the approach to physical therapy treatment programs in this area comes from a perspective that primarily emphasizes neurophysiologic concepts.[10, 14, 23] In this chapter I diverge from this point of view and suggest that the emerging science of motor behavior has been essentially ignored by the physical therapist. Kelso[24] suggests that "a full understanding of human movement . . . . can only come about if we integrate behavioral work (which tends to focus on the outcome of performance) with kinesiology (which provides us with information about the kinematics of human movement) and neurophysiology (which tells us the nature of the underlying neural mechanisms involved in controlled movement)." Theoretical perspectives are discussed and empirical evidence presented from human movement research and the literature on motor learning, in particular that which has relevance to movement reeducation programs for subjects recovering from a cerebral vascular accident.

I have chosen to focus upon two major motor learning issues relevant to stroke rehabilitation. The first centers upon the use of intrinsic and extrinsic feedback to facilitate motor learning, and the second emphasizes recent views regarding the structuring of the practice or, in this case, the treatment session.

INTRINSIC AND EXTRINSIC FEEDBACK

Aside from practice itself, feedback is considered one of the most powerful variables affecting motor learning.[40] Feedback can be either intrinsic or extrinsic in origin. Intrinsic feedback is *inherent* sensory information that comes from the specialized receptors in muscle, joint, tendon, and skin as well as that from visual and auditory receptors either during or following movement production.[40] In contrast, extrinsic feedback is *augmented* information about movement provided to the performer from an external source. One form of extrinsic feedback is knowledge of results (KR) and is defined as information about the response outcome.[32] Salmoni and associates[38] suggest that KR must also be at least verbalizable. This distinguishes it from merely seeing one's response outcome. Because seeing is influenced by perceptual and attentional variables, it would be difficult to define exactly what constituted the KR. Instead, KR, in a strict sense, is defined as verbal, post-response, augmented feedback about the response outcome.

Another type of extrinsic feedback is knowledge of performance (KP) (see Gentile[17] for a review). In contrast to KR, KP is information about the movement pattern produced, rather than the outcome.[40] Here we assume that the principles derived from experimental studies relevant to the function of KR are the same for KP. At least, there is no evidence at the present time to suggest otherwise. Magill[32] refers to KP as information about what caused the response outcome. The goal response must be well defined in order to differentiate KR and KP. In the following gait training example, the goal response is a longer stance period or, more precisely, a right left stance ratio approaching unity. When I say, "Stance time on the right leg was too short," I am providing KR. If instead, I say, "Weight shift onto the right leg during stance was inadequate," I am providing KP, because it was the inadequate weight shift onto the right leg that was primarily responsible for the short stance time.

In the therapeutic setting, KP is used more often, while KR has been primarily used in the experimental laboratory. The use of KP is more appropriate in the therapeutic setting for two reasons. First, the outcome (KR) is often obvious to the patient, while the movement response that caused the outcome is not so obvious and may need to be supplied by the therapist. For example, during transfer training, if the patient needed assistance coming to a standing position, it is obvious that independent standing was not achieved. The therapist augments the outcome information when suggesting that the patient did not lean forward enough prior to the standing attempt. The second reason KP is most often used in the therapeutic setting is that there are often several components to the desired movement outcome. This is contrasted with the experimental setting, where for simplicity the response outcome and the pattern of the response are often one and the same. In other words, in the therapy arena, there are many potential variables that need to be constrained in order for the appropriate outcome to occur. The learner acquires the capability to control the many "degrees of freedom," a term used by motor learning researchers that refers to the many variables of a movement response.[24] The therapist can focus the patient's attention on the critical components of the response outcome by using appropriate KP.

In the stroke patient, intrinsic feedback is often distorted or, in severe cases, absent.[44] The common viewpoint suggests that this deficit amplifies the apparent need for appropriate extrinsic feedback. For example, impaired position sense can interfere with limb placement during stair climbing. Extrinsic feedback, such as verbal cuing provided at the appropriate time, can effect more normal positioning of the affected limb. On the other hand, if the patient has intact position sense but impaired motor control, then the extrinsic feedback might direct his attention to the inherent feedback. Thus, the therapist can use extrinsic feedback to both augment impaired intrinsic feedback mechanisms or to direct conscious attention to inherent feedback cues.

Both intrinsic and extrinsic feedback are emphasized in the many physical therapeutic techniques employed in stroke rehabilitation. Sullivan 'and co-workers[45] state, "Visual input is one of the most important elements a therapist can use in treatment." Carr and Shepherd[11] suggest that the therapist relay to the patient "information about muscle contraction immediately as it occurs." Herman[20] emphasizes that the brain-damaged person would relearn more effective motor control if he were given continuous accurate feedback. It is clear that intrinsic and extrinsic feedback are believed to be powerful variables for enhancing motor relearning.

EXTRINSIC FEEDBACK AND MOTOR LEARNING

Extrinsic feedback can be thought of as functioning in several different capacities with respect to motor learning.[3] First, and perhaps most important, it provides information to the performer about response outcome and error. A motor task can be viewed as a problem that the performer must solve. Augmented feedback provides information relevant to the solution of the problem. In fact, early researchers showed that human subjects use KR to correct errors on the next response.[15] Second, extrinsic feedback can function as a reinforcement or reward for a given behavior. This is particularly true as the performance approaches the goal movement with practice. Third, extrinsic feedback has been described as motivational[31] as it relates to goal achievement. It has also been viewed as a form of guidance that directs the performer toward a desired outcome and "energizes" the learner.[38] When KR is used, subjects tend to practice longer, try harder, and stay interested in the task longer than when KR is not used.[5, 12]

Theoretical perspectives hold that extrinsic feedback is critical to the establishment of an internal reference of correctness.[2, 40] There is evidence to suggest that this internal reference of correctness develops with practice, and one interpretation is that it can take the place of intrinsic feedback to the extent that performance is maintained.[40] This is the essential process by which the use of extrinsic feedback can facilitate motor learning.

LEARNING VS. PERFORMANCE

Learning is not directly observable.[32] It is defined as a relatively permanent change in the capability for responding that results from practice or experience.[40] The essence of a "relatively permanent change" is that quality which distinguishes learning from a more temporary change in behavior that does not persist with time. A clever analogy was offered by Schmidt.[40] When water freezes, it becomes ice, but this is only a temporary change that is reversible once I remove the ice from the freezer. On the other hand, when an egg is boiled, it becomes hard, and this metamorphosis is not reversible, that is, the change is relatively permanent regardless of where I put the egg.

In therapeutic settings, performance effects, like the transitory effects seen in the ice cube, are too often confused with learning. If the learning goal is to perform the motor activity without extrinsic feedback, one way to distinguish performance effects from learning is to evaluate the acquired behavior without the practice variable. For example, KP is a practice variable that is used during treatment to facilitate a desired response. If the response is obtained in the presence of KP, all that can be said is that there is a change in performance. A meaningful test comes from demonstrating the same change in performance when the extrinsic feedback is withdrawn.

CLOSED- AND OPEN-LOOP CONTROL AND MOTOR LEARNING

The use of intrinsic and extrinsic feedback differs with respect to whether or not the movement is controlled primarily by open- or closed-loop processes. A critical difference between closed- and open-loop models of movement control is that closed-loop models rely on incoming feedback to determine the response, while open-loop models do not. Open-loop models are referred to by some as motor programs that contain the necessary temporal and quantitative elements of the desired movement response.[40] Closed-loop control systems are often referred to as servomechanisms or self-regulating systems utilizing feedback, error detection, and correction.[40] There is, however, considerable evidence to suggest that some motions can be executed quite well without on-line use of feedback.[8, 25–27, 37, 46] Furthermore, it has been suggested that well-learned motions, like a practiced gymnastics routine, do not rely upon the conscious processing of incoming feedback to control the response. Hellenbrandt[19] states that a "specific technique being learned is considered maximally efficient when it runs its course automatically." It should not be interpreted that feedback is not used in these cases, but that it may be handled more automatically, i.e., at a less conscious level of the nervous system.[11, 35] Recently, in contrast to feedback mechanisms, feedforward mechanisms have been implicated in motor learning.[1]

THEORETICAL PERSPECTIVES OF MOTOR LEARNING

Originally, Adams'[2] closed-loop theory of motor learning proposed the existence of two separate memory constructs: the memory trace and the perceptual trace. The memory trace was responsible for movement initiation, while the perceptual trace was responsible for guiding the limb, once initiated, to the target position. Adams postulated that the strength of the perceptual trace was directly related to the quantity of KR provided during the practice period. From Adams' perspective, the ability to consistently perform the acquired goal movement depends upon the strength of the perceptual trace.

Schmidt's[39] schema theory relies heavily upon open-loop processes, which are thought to be primarily responsible for the execution of fast or ballistic responses. A schema is an abstract memory construct that represents a rule or generalization about an event, perception, or motor action. It is the basis of the schema theory of discrete motor learning[39] and represents an abstract relation formed from experience within a particular class of movements. For example, I have had experience rolling a bowling ball. My memory for this task is a general rule representing the relation of my performance at this task with the action commands and my sensations associated with the activity. I do not necessarily have a memory (or perceptual trace) for every time I rolled a bowling ball, but I do have a generalized rule that is abstracted from my experience.

Because Schmidt's theory is concerned with open-loop control processes, the concept of the motor program is central to its understanding. Schmidt's definition of a motor program takes into account the fact that very fast feedback loops, such as the monosynaptic stretch reflex loop, can and do operate during responses and are capable of corrections and small modifications that enable preservation of the desired response. On the contrary, such preservative feedback responses are *not* capable of changing the goal response or *selecting* another set of commands. Therefore, "a motor program is an abstract structure in memory that is prepared in advance of the movement; when it is executed, the result is the contraction and relaxation of muscles causing movement to occur without the involvement of feedback leading to corrections for errors in selection."[41] In other words, selecting another set of commands involves less automatic (i.e., closed-loop) processes.

In fact, schema theory suggests that the motor program is a

generalized prestructured plan that is parameterized according to the specific task demands. For example, I have a generalized motor program for rolling a bowling ball. Depending upon the specific situation, I will select specific parameters such as force and direction, which specify the particular roll at that time. How do I know which parameters to select for which response? When I am first learning, I am not sure, and I make errors (i.e., bowl a gutter ball!), but with practice, I am able to select the appropriate parameters for the desired response. How does the learner develop an association between the appropriate parameters and the desired response? This question is relevant to the physical therapist, who must assist the patient through this process during neuromuscular rehabilitation.

Schema theory supports a strong role for extrinsic feedback in motor learning. Specifically, there are four essential features related to the motor response that the performer uses when learning. Figure 4–1 illustrates the relevant relationships between (a) the initial conditions before the movement, (b) which parameters or motor commands (i.e., response specification) were assigned to the generalized motor program, (c) the actual consequences of the movement in the form of extrinsic feedback, and (d) the actual intrinsic sensory feedback from the response. These critical features are used to establish the abstract rules or schema. There are actually two schema derived from these relevant features. The first is the recall schema, which is responsible for movement production and is analogous to Adams' memory trace. The recall schema is the abstract rule that defines the relation between the response parameters specified and the actual movement produced. The next is the recognition schema, which is responsible for response evaluation and is analogous to Adams' perceptual trace. The recognition schema is the abstract rule that defines the relation between the sensory consequences (i.e., intrinsic sensory cues) and the actual movement produced.

The essential feature of Schmidt's theory is the development of rules that relate response parameters and associated sensory consequences to actual responses. From this, it is clear that knowledge about the actual response outcome (i.e., provided through extrinsic feedback) is essential to the development of the rules. Schmidt[40] states that, "Responses for which any of the four stored elements are missing will result in degraded

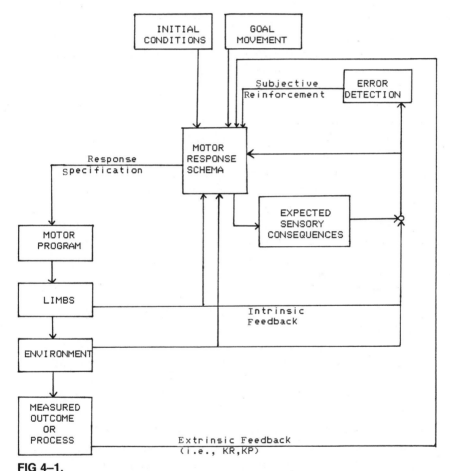

FIG 4–1.
The motor response schema with respect to the initial conditions, response specifications, and intrinsic and extrinsic feedback for one trial (the recall and recognition schemas are combined for clarity. *KR,* knowledge of results; *KP,* knowledge of performance (Adapted from Schmidt RA: A schema theory of discrete motor skill learning. *Psychol Rev* 1975; 82:225–260.)

learning of the rules." This has particular relevance to the stroke victim who has distortions in response activation[36] and sensory consequences.[44] Thus, the old rules developed prior to the stroke may not be representative of the poststroke relationships. New rules will need to be established in the process of motor relearning.

For example, the response parameters for reaching forward and grasping a cup are associated with certain initial conditions related to the position of the arm and the cup. A given force of contractions generated at the appropriate times are associated with the successful completion of the activity. In addition, the expected sensory consequences are associated with a particular movement outcome. These relationships presumably change following a cardiovascular accident. The previously used parameters are inadequate as a result of abnormal movement synergies and inadequate muscle force generation. In addition, the expected sensory consequences are no longer useful because of changes in the ability to monitor ongoing sensory information or interpret postresponse sensory information. Thus, new relationships will need to be developed associating the existing parameter capabilities with movement outcome, and the new sensory consequences will need to be associated with movement outcome. In other words, a transformation of the previous relationships must be facilitated with the use of appropriate extrinsic feedback.

Schema theory predicts that rule strength depends on the subject's experience pairing response parameters with actual responses for movements within the same response class. Particularly, rule strength is a function of both (a) the amount of experience pairing a given response with its associated response parameters and (b) experience with different responses within the same response class. Thus, if I make an error in response specification (i.e., choose the wrong parameter) such as choosing too much force, my actual outcome (KR) will have been to overshoot the target, but this variability gives me additional useful information about the abstract relationship between response specification and movement outcome. By this logic, errors are not detrimental to learning, but rather, they can provide valuable information for rule abstraction, if extrinsic feedback is provided. This has important implications in the therapeutic setting. Schema theory postulates that errors and variability within a response class are beneficial to rule development. Therefore, patient errors can facilitate rule development when they are accompanied by KR and/or KP.

Both Adam's and Schmidt's theories regard intrinsic and extrinsic feedback as important for motor learning. Further, both theories provide for the establishment of an internal reference of correctness that can be used to identify errors either during the movement, as in closed-loop control, or prior to the next response, as in open-loop control. Thus, it follows that both theories suggest that, with appropriate practice, the correct response can be made without extrinsic feedback. The specific differences between the two theories are centered on the memory representation of the movement. Adam's theory suggests that each movement response is stored as a trace, while Schmidt suggests that the specific response parameters of a desired movement response are stored as an abstracted rule. In addition, Adams' theory is limited to closed-loop, slow positioning responses, while Schmidt's theory can be used to explain both open-loop fast responses, which are primarily governed by motor programs, as well as slow responses.

THERAPEUTIC IMPLICATIONS OF OPEN- AND CLOSED-LOOP PROCESSES

It is relevant that open and closed-loop control mechanisms appear to make use of conscious feedback quite differently. Conscious utilization of feedback is attributed to closed-loop processes, but not open-loop processes. It follows that if the desired response is more "open-loop," a treatment approach that persists in emphasizing the conscious utilization of continuous feedback during the response may be inappropriate. For example, when I walk, I do not think about dorsiflexing my ankle during swing phase, nor do I watch my feet with every step. Instead, it is highly likely that central mechanisms are responsible for coordinating the ongoing response.[18] This central control is considered analogous to open-loop processes. In contrast, when I trace a line onto tracing paper, I pay attention to visual information and guide my pen with that information in order to remain on target and reduce my error. This control is best represented by closed-loop processes. From a therapeutic perspective, while it would be appropriate to emphasize the continuous conscious use of visual feedback during a task primarily under closed-loop control, this approach would not be appropriate for the performance of a task that was primarily controlled by open-loop processes. Thus, the therapeutic effectiveness of intrinsic and extrinsic feedback may be determined by the level of ongoing conscious feedback utilization required by the particular goal movement.

USING FEEDBACK TO PROMOTE MOTOR LEARNING

Clearly, motor learning theories[2, 39] and the therapeutic literature[10, 11, 14, 45] stress that utilization of intrinsic and extrinsic feedback during practice will facilitate learning. While the therapist can direct attention to the patient's intrinsic feedback, such feedback, because of its inherent nature, cannot be directly manipulated. Therefore, this discussion will center on three major ways that extrinsic feedback can be used to facilitate motor learning.

Although there are many ways to vary the amount of extrinsic feedback, this discussion will emphasize three major variations. Variations can occur in (a) the total number of exposures to the information presented across all practice sessions (absolute frequency), (b) the percentage of exposures given within a single practice session (expressed as relative frequency), and (c) the number of different sensory channels through which information is provided. For example, if KR and/or KP are provided on every other trial of a 20-trial practice session, the absolute frequency is ten exposures, while the relative frequency is 50%. The amount of extrinsic feedback can be increased by allowing more practice sessions and thereby increasing the absolute frequency, or by providing information more frequently within the practice session, thereby increasing the relative frequency. In addition, the amount of extrinsic feedback can be increased by providing it through more sensory channels, such as the auditory, visual, and proprioceptive systems.

Theoretically, the more exposures to intrinsic and extrinsic feedback, and the more modes through which it is provided, the stronger will become the internal reference of correctness (or recognition schema) as well as the internal movement program (or recall schema). Adams and associates[4] compared groups given enriched feedback and diminished feedback and found, in a no-KR transfer condition, that the group having experienced the enriched feedback demonstrated less error than the group with diminished feedback provided the feedback conditions were the same in acquisition and transfer. In a recent study examining different modes of sensory feedback, Mulder and Hulstyn[34] similarly found that subjects who received both natural (proprioceptive, visual, and tactile) and artificial (electromyographic and force) feedback during training demonstrated more range of motion during a test than subjects who just received natural feedback. These results are not really surprising.

In contrast, motor learning experiments that have examined the effects of different relative frequency feedback schedules on motor learning seem to be equivocal. These studies show superior performance during the practice trials for those subjects with high, as compared with low, relative frequency feedback schedules; but in a no-KR retention test, the tendency was for groups that practiced at low relative frequency schedules to perform with less error and more consistency than the groups which practiced at high relative frequency schedules.[6, 22, 47]

In addition, recent research[48] has led to the hypothesis that

there is an optimum relative frequency schedule that will promote motor learning as measured in a nonextrinsic feedback
transfer test. Too little (i.e., 10%) is detrimental in that a coherent relation between the action plan and actual movement
production is never recognized, while too much (i.e., 100%)
may foster dependency (see Salmoni et al.[38] for a discussion)
on the KR/KP such that the subject has less need to utilize the
intrinsic proprioceptive cues inherent in the performance. If
learning is based partially on the development of an internal
reference of correctness, and subsequent error detection
mechanism, dependency upon extrinsic feedback may detract
from the development of such internal relationships.

From the viewpoint of relative frequency, schedules with
more frequent extrinsic feedback presentations are good for
performance, but could be detrimental to learning. It is clear
that more research is needed in order to establish an understanding of appropriate extrinsic feedback practice schedules
and their relation to the learning goals. For now, we should
not so readily accept the notion that practice schedules with
high relative frequencies are the best for neuromuscular relearning. Suggestions to use continuous extrinsic feedback during treatment may lead to dependence upon that feedback and
a false sense of "learning" rather than the development of in-
dependence necessary for performance in the absence of these
extrinsic feedback cues.

STAGES OF MOTOR LEARNING AND EXTRINSIC FEEDBACK

Fitts and Posner[16] describe three stages of motor learning.
The first of these stages is labelled the cognitive stage, because
much of the emphasis is on conscious processing of the task
requirements. Performance during this stage is full of errors
and highly variable. For example, when I learned how to operate a manual transmission, I had to think about the position
in which to put the gear shift, when to push down on the
clutch and when to release the clutch. I often stalled the car

or ground the gears. During this first stage, the performer has a vague sense of the problem, but is unsure of what needs to be done to correct the response. Guidance during this stage can effect marked improvements in performance. My friend said, "Ready, clutch in, gas off, shift, clutch out, and gas on . . . ." This helped me successfully complete the gear shift without stalling the engine.

The next stage is marked by the beginning of the development of an internal reference of correctness and associated internal movement program. This second stage is called the associative stage. Performance is less variable and more accurate. Attention is shifted from the gross task requirements to finer details. I can remember thinking about how to make a smooth transition between the shift and the acceleration of the car once I felt comfortable about the general shifting procedure.

The last stage, called the autonomous stage, is characterized by minimal attention to the performance. Full error-detection capabilities have developed, and performance is very stable. Once I had "learned" to operate a manual transmission, I could attend to other things, such as listen to the radio or talk to a passenger, and still be able to perform my shifting smoothly and without error.

Within a therapeutic context, the patient initially needs strong guidance during the cognitive stage. For example, when teaching a wheelchair transfer, verbal guidance regarding the procedure (i.e., lock brakes, lift up footrests, position feet on floor, scoot forward . . . etc.) will facilitate the performance of the task. Progression to the associative stage can be effected by providing less verbal guidance and allowing the patient to begin forming the appropriate associations between the action plan and the inherent sensory consequences. Here error information should be provided when necessary, but the patient should also be allowed to develop their own error-detection mechanism. Finally, progression to the automatic stage is evident when the task can be performed in a more distracting environment. Here, performance of the task has become more automatic, given that attention may be allocated to more than just the immediate activity. Fitts and Posner[16] discuss the similarity between a well-learned performance and a reflex. Neither requires any conscious attention.

BIOFEEDBACK AS A FORM OF AUGMENTED FEEDBACK

Biofeedback can be considered a type of extrinsic feedback.[40] By definition, it is more a form of KP than KR. It is a term coined in 1969 to mean "the use of instrumentation to make covert physiological processes more overt to the patient."[49] Visual and auditory electromyographic biofeedback has been shown to be an effective method for training subjects to consciously control the recruitment and firing frequency of single motor units.[7] Although the literature reviewed seems to emphasize the performance effects, that is, with biofeedback present, Basmajian[7] states that, "Some persons can be trained to gain control of isolated motor units . . . with both visual and aural cues shut off. . . ." However, this latter process seems to involve a certain amount of concentration.

In a recent review of electromyographic biofeedback application to stroke patients, Wolf[49] stated that "although EMG biofeedback may augment movement capabilities at least as well as an exercise regimen, data relating neuromuscular changes to function are limited." Wolf asks if a "significant increase in active ankle dorsiflexion range of motion following (bio)feedback training means that the hemiplegic walks better." I would speculate that it does not, necessarily, for the following reason. Gait is undoubtedly centrally generated[18] and relies minimally upon any conscious attention to specific muscular feedback information.

The emphasis in electromyographic biofeedback training is to bring the normally unconscious control of specific muscles under conscious control. This clearly is analogous to the cognitive stage described by Fitts and Posner.[16] The question is, first, how do we then facilitate the patient's progress into the automatic stage, that stage that represents the well-learned response (i.e., without biofeedback)? And second, how do we facilitate the use of a specific response in a functional activity? Perhaps the development of training protocols that deemphasize the more closed-loop, conscious control of motion while emphasizing the more open-loop, unconscious, automatic control necessary for functional activity, will prove effective. The use of a progressively intermittent biofeedback schedule seems like a logical first step toward this aim, but this is certainly not a closed issue; further research is necessary.

In summary, evidence was presented demonstrating that, in general, extrinsic feedback facilitates motor learning. In contrast, increasing the relative frequency of extrinsic feedback within a practice session does not necessarily lead to improved performance on a no-KR/KP transfer test over levels of low relative frequency. In fact, there is a suggestion that conditions of high relative frequency, although beneficial to motor performance, are detrimental to motor learning as measured in a no-extrinsic feedback retention test. Finally, electromyographic biofeedback was discussed with regard to open- and closed-loop control models. While conscious control of specific muscles might be appropriate during the early cognitive stage of motor learning, such closed-loop control is not appropriate for later, more automatic stages of motor learning.

STRUCTURING THE PRACTICE SESSION DURING TREATMENT

VARIABILITY IN PRACTICE

An important prediction from schema theory was that rule development is facilitated by multiple and variable experience with the particular class of movements controlled by a given generalized motor program. For example, as I develop a recall schema for rolling a bowling ball, if I have experience bowling to various pin arrangements, I will develop a stronger rule relating the selected force parameters and desired outcome than if I only practice bowling to one pin arrangement. In short, schema theory predicts that variable practice within a class of movements will facilitate skill transfer to a novel condition over constant practice. This prediction generated a tremendous number of empirical studies.

In reviewing these studies, Shapiro and Schmidt[42] found only minimal support for variability in practice in the adult, but strong support for it with children (see Lee et al.[30] for a more recent review). One explanation offered for this discrepancy is that children's recall schemata are more prone to the influence of variability, because their schemata are not well developed, while the adult already has a well-developed rule, especially for the kinds of tasks used in these studies. The adult's schemata are much less prone to the influence of additional variability.

How does variability in practice relate to the rehabilitation of the stroke victim? Earlier, it was suggested that the stroke patient has, by virtue of the neurologic lesion, distortions in both response activation and sensory feedback. In light of these changes, the old rules are ineffective. It seems likely that new rules, or modifications of old rules, representing the new relations between response specifications and outcome (recall) and sensory consequences and outcome (recognition) will need to be developed during the motor relearning phase. In a sense, then, the stroke patient is similar to the child who has less well-developed rules than the adult. The stroke patient has a well-developed set of rules, but these rules are no longer effective. The rehabilitation treatment program can be viewed as an opportunity to facilitate the development of new or modified rules. This is one place where the notion of variability in practice may be relevant.

For example, when teaching the patient how to stand up from a chair, I can introduce variability by changing the height of the chair from trial to trial, or I can vary the terrain during gait training from a smooth waxed floor to an uneven gravel walkway. The rationale here is to allow the patient to experience the various force and postural requirements necessary to achieve the goal. In the future, the patient who has experienced this variable practice should be more likely to choose the proper force and postural parameters to stand from an unknown chair or walk on an unfamiliar terrain than the patient who has always practiced from the same chair or walked on the same surface. Notice that both these patients may appear to perform well in the typical rehabilitation setting, but the prediction is that the one who received variable practice has greater potential for success after discharge into a different environment than the one who received constant practice.

INTRATASK AND INTERTASK ORGANIZATION

Consideration of both intratask and intertask organization is important in structuring the practice session. Is there an optimum organization that facilitates recall and transfer of motor learning? We know that in general a treatment session might consist of transfer training, bed mobility, gait training, and neuromuscular facilitation and reeducation. However, little attention has been focused on how movement goals are best organized within an activity or how these various activities are best organized within a treatment session. Some schools of thought support a developmental sequence approach[10, 23] to intertask organization. However, there is no empirical evidence to suggest that this approach is more beneficial than any other approach.

There are several theoretical perspectives in the fields of verbal and motor learning and memory that suggest that certain intertask organizations facilitate recall and transfer of motor skills. The spacing of repeated items to be learned has been shown to be critical for recall.[9, 33] Specifically, Melton[33] found that the probability of recall of items (words) twice presented in a word list, increases as the number of interpolated words between its presentations increases. This counterintuitive observation became known as the repetition or spacing effect.[21] The analogy in motor skills is blocked vs. random practice orders, which contrasts zero spacing between repetitions (blocked practice) with all spacings greater than zero (random practice). For example, a blocked practice order might consist of a series of standing-pivot transfers followed by a series of other activities and then a repetition of the standing-pivot transfer. The spacing effect suggests that a random practice order facilitates motor recall over a blocked practice order.[43]

Motor learning researchers manipulate the intratask and intertask practice orders and examine the effects on motor recall. Practice orders are designated as random, serial, or blocked. Given that A, B, and C are three different tasks: random (i.e., nonrepeating, unpredictable order, such as ACBCAB) or serial (i.e., predictable order, but not repeated, such as ABCABC) order practice is compared with blocked order practice (i.e., repeating, predictable order, such as AAAAAA). Recent experimental evidence that investigated the effects of practice order suggests, counterintuitively, that if the practice order is random or serial, recall and transfer of motor skills are facilitated over blocked order practice.[28, 43]

Some human learning and memory researchers postulate that the facilitation of recall obtained in the practice order paradigm is due to certain cognitive processes.[13, 29] Assume that each practice attempt of the task is like a problem that the performer must solve. He must organize an action plan.[32] If the practice order is blocked, the performer can remember the action plan from the previous attempt and select it again, without having to generate it again. However, if the practice order is random or serial, a new action plan must be generated each time. When the original task is repeated after the interpolated tasks, the previously used plan has been forgotten, or at least it is not as easily accessible; therefore, the plan must be regenerated. It is suggested that the process of generating the plan on subsequent attempts is what ultimately facilitates recall of the task.[13, 28, 29]

How do these practice order effects relate to the structuring of a physical therapy treatment session? They suggest that a random or serial intertask ordering of activities within one treatment session would be more beneficial for eventual recall and transfer than repeatedly practicing one activity per treatment session. In other words, I could organize my treatment session on an intertask level around a series of transfers, followed by facilitation and reeducation, followed by gait training, and could repeat this sequence several times within one half-hour treatment session. Further, consideration of the intratask context is relevant. Practice order effects would suggest that incorporating specific movements (i.e., elbow extension) within a functional context, such as reaching for an object, would facilitate motor learning over practice of the movement task in an isolated nonfunctional context.

In summary, recent experimental evidence has been presented relevant to the practical structuring of the therapeutic treatment session. It has been suggested that practice variability, that is, practicing several variations of a task, will facilitate transfer of that task to a novel situation. Further, nonrepetitive intertask practice orders and functional intratask contexts may facilitate recall and transfer of motor skills. There is probably a preferential practice structure that facilitates recall and transfer of motor skills, and this structure may vary between healthy and disabled populations. Certainly, further research is needed to examine these issues in the rehabilitation context.

SUMMARY

It was suggested earlier that research in the field of motor behavior has much to offer the physical therapist. This chapter has provided a global framework of motor performance and learning, within which the use of feedback and the structure of the treatment session were discussed. The essential elements of the literature reviewed can be used in the design and implementation of physical therapy programs in which motor relearning is an important goal.

Augmented feedback in the form of KR, KP, or biofeedback, if used appropriately, can facilitate the development of both an internal reference of correctness and internal response mechanisms essential to motor learning. Given this perspective about the significance of feedback, the importance of relative-frequency feedback schedules, stage of motor learning, and the goal movement task were emphasized. With respect to structuring the therapy session, task ordering within and between tasks was emphasized.

A distinction between motor performance and learning is critical to the intelligent use of feedback variations and the efficient structuring of the treatment session. Given that, in most instances, motor learning is the primary goal, the following considerations are suggested for treatment planning:

1. The selection of the appropriate sensory channels through which extrinsic feedback is provided will depend upon the evaluation findings. While the use of more channels seems desirable, the amount of feedback provided should probably depend upon the stage of motor learning. The early cognitive stage requires strong guidance, while the associative stage is marked by less guidance to allow the patient to develop the internal relationships of action and sensory consequences. Too much feedback during this stage, while beneficial to immediate performance, may be detrimental to later performance in the absence of extrinsic feedback cues. The final automatic stage of motor learning is marked by little conscious attention to the task (and little is known about this).

2. While high relative frequency feedback schedules are beneficial to performance, they may promote dependency on extrinsic feedback and deter the development of internal mechanisms that allow the learner to produce effective responses and/or to evaluate their correctness. Progression to lower relative frequency feedback schedules is desirable to promote performance outside the practice context, where extrinsic feedback is not always available.

3. The type of movement task must be considered with respect to the conscious use of feedback. Open-loop, controlled responses utilize predominantly postresponse error information, while closed-loop movements mainly utilize error information during response execution.

4. Practicing variations of the movement task seems to pro-

mote transfer of motor skills to novel movement variations to a greater extent than constant practice of the same movement.

5. While a repetitive task practice schedule may seem beneficial to performance, a nonrepetitive task practice schedule appears to promote later recall of the desired response.

ACKNOWLEDGEMENT

I would like to express my appreciation to Elizabeth R. Gardner, R.P.T., Rebecca Lewthwaite, Ph.D., and Richard A. Schmidt, Ph.D. for helpful suggestions on an earlier draft of this chapter.

REFERENCES

1. Abbs JH, Greco VL, Cole KJ: Control of multimovement coordination: Sensorimotor mechanisms in speech motor programming. *J Mot Behav* 1984; 16:195–232.
2. Adams JA: A closed-loop theory of motor learning. *J Mot Behav* 1971; 3:111–149.
3. Adams JA: Theoretical issues for knowledge of results, in Stelmach GE (ed): *Information Processing in Motor Control and Learning.* San Francisco, Academic Press, 1978, pp 229–240.
4. Adams JA, Goetz ET, Marshall PH: Response feedback and motor learning. *J Exp Psychol* 1972; 92:391–397.
5. Arps GF: Work with KR versus work without KR. *Psychol Monographs* 1920; 28 (No 125).
6. Baird IS, Hughes GH: Effects of frequency and specificity of information feedback on the acquisition and extinction of a positioning task. *Percep Mot Skills* 1972; 34:567–572.
7. Basmajian JV: *Muscles Alive.* Baltimore, Williams & Wilkins Co, 1974.
8. Bizzi E, Polit A: Processes controlling visually evoked movements. *Neuropsychologia* 1979; 17:203–213.
9. Bjork RA, Allen TW: The spacing effect; Consolidation or differential encoding. *J Verbal Learn Verbal Behav* 1970; 9:567–572.
10. Bobath B: *Adult Hemiplegia: Evaluation and Treatment.* London, William Heinemann Medical Books Ltd, 1978.
11. Carr JH, Shepherd RB: *A Motor Relearning Program for Stroke.* Rockville, Md, Aspen Systems Corp, 1983.

12. Crawley SL: An experimental investigation of recovery from work. *Arch Psychol* 1926; 13:26.
13. Cuddy LJ, Jacoby LL: When forgetting helps memory: An analysis of repetition effects. *J Verbal Learn Verbal Behav* 1982; 21:451–467.
14. Davies PM: *Steps to Follow: A Guide to the Treatment of Adult Hemiplegia.* New York, Springer-Verlag, 1985.
15. Elwell JL, Grindley GC: The effect of knowledge of results on learning and performance. *Br J Psychol* 1938; 29:39–54.
16. Fitts PM, Posner MI: *Human Performance.* Belmont, Calif., Brooks/Cole, 1967.
17. Gentile AM: A Working model of skill acquisition with application to teaching. *Quest* 1972; 17:3–23.
18. Grillner S: Control of locomotion in bipeds, tetrapods, and fish, in Brooks VB (ed): *Handbook of Physiology.* Baltimore: Williams & Wilkins Co, 1981, vol 2, pp 1179–1236.
19. Hellenbrandt FA: Motor learning reconsidered: A study of change, in Payton OD, Hirt S, Newton RA (eds): *Scientific Bases for Neurophysiologic Approaches to Therapeutic Exercise.* Philadelphia, FA Davis Co, 1978, pp 33–45.
20. Herman R: Augmented sensory feedback in the control of limb movement, in Fields WS (ed): *Neural Organization and its Relevance to Prosthetics.* New York, Intercontinental Medical Book Corp, 1973, pp 197–212.
21. Hintzman DL: Theoretical implications of the spacing effect, in Solso RL (ed): *Theories in Cognitive Psychology: The Loyola Symposium.* Potomac, Md, Erlbaum, 1974, pp 77–99.
22. Ho L, Shea JB: Effects of relative frequency of knowledge of results on retention of a motor skill. *Percept Mot Skills* 1978; 46:859–866.
23. Johnstone M: *Restoration of Motor Function in the Stroke Patient.* London, Churchill Livingstone, 1978.
24. Kelso JAS: The process approach to understanding human motor behavior: An introduction, in Kelso JAS (ed): *Human Motor Behavior: An Introduction.* Hillsdale, NJ, Lawrence Erlbaum Assoc Pub, 1982, pp 3–19.
25. Kelso JAS, Holt KG: Exploring a vibratory systems analysis of human movement production. *J Neurophysiol* 1980; 43:1183–1196.
26. Kelso JAS, Holt KG, Flatt AE: The role of proprioception in the

perception and control of human movement: Toward a theoretical reassessment. *Percep Psychophys* 1980; 28:45–52.

27. Lashley KS: The accuracy of movement in the absence of excitation from the moving organ. *Am J Physiol* 1917; 43:169–194.

28. Lee TD, Magill RA: The locus of contextual interference in motor-skill acquisition. *J Exp Psychol Learn Mem Cogn* 1983; 9:730–746.

29. Lee TD, Magill RA: Can forgetting facilitate skill acquisition? in Goodman D, Wilberg RB, Franks IM (eds): *Differing Perspectives in Motor Learning, Memory, and Control.* New York, North-Holland, 1985, pp 3–22.

30. Lee TD, Magill RA, Weeks DJ: Influence of practice schedule on testing schema theory predictions in adults. *J Mot Behav* 1985; 17:283–299.

31. Locke EA, Cartledge N, Koeppel J: Motivational effects of knowledge of results: A goal-setting phenomenon. *Psychol Bull* 1968; 70:474–485.

32. Magill RA: *Motor Learning Concepts and Application.* Dubuque, Ia, William C Brown Pub, 1985.

33. Melton AW: Repetition and retrieval from memory. *Science* 1967; 158:532.

34. Mulder T, Hulstijn W: Sensory feedback in the learning of a novel motor task. *J Mot Behav* 1985; 17:110–128.

35. Mulder T, Hulstyn W: Sensory feedback therapy and theoretical knowledge of motor control and learning. *Am J Phys Med* 1984; 63:226–244.

36. Nakamura R, Taniguchi R: Reaction time in patients with cerebral hemiparesis. *Neuropsychologia* 1977; 15:845–848.

37. Polit A, Bizzi A: Characteristics of motor programs underlying arm movements in monkeys. *J Neurophysiol* 1979; 42:183–194.

38. Salmoni AW, Schmidt RA, Walter CB: Knowledge of results and motor learning: A review and critical reappraisal. *Psychol Bull* 1984; 95:355–386.

39. Schmidt RA: A schema theory of discrete motor skill learning. *Psychol Rev* 1975; 82:225–260.

40. Schmidt RA: *Motor Control and Learning.* Champaign, Ill, Human Kinetics Pub, Inc, 1982.

41. Schmidt RA: More on motor programs, in Kelso JAS (ed): *Human Motor Behavior: An Introduction.* Hillsdale, NJ, Lawrence Erlbaum Assoc Pub, 1982, pp 189–217.

42. Shapiro DC, Schmidt RA: The schema theory: Recent evidence and developmental implications, in Kelso JAS, Clark JE (eds): *The Development of Movement Control and Coordination.* New York, John Wiley & Sons, 1982, pp 113–150.
43. Shea JB, Morgan RL: Contextual interference effects on the acquisition, retention and transfer of a motor skill. *J Exp Psychol Hum Learn Mem* 1979; 5:179–187.
44. Smith DL, Akhtar AJ, Garraway WM: Proprioception and spatial neglect after stroke. *Age Ageing* 1982; 12:63–69.
45. Sullivan RE, Markos PD, Minor MD: *An Integrated Approach to Therapeutic Exercise Theory and Clinical Application.* Reston, Va, Reston Pub Co, 1982.
46. Taub E, Berman AJ: Movement and learning in the absence of sensory feedback, in Freedman SJ (ed): *The Neuropsychology of Spatially Oriented Behavior.* Homewood, Ill, Dorsey Press, 1968, pp 173–192.
47. Taylor A, Noble CE: Acquisition and extinction phenomena in human trial-and-error learning under different schedules of reinforcing feedback. *Percep Mot Skills* 1962; 15:31–44.
48. Winstein C, Schmidt RA: Effect of knowledge of performance on the acquisition of a spatial-temporal movement pattern. Poster presentation at the North American Society for the Psychology of Sport and Physical Activity, Annual Conference, Gulfport, Miss, May 1985.
49. Wolf SI: Electromyographic biofeedback applications to stroke patients. *Phys Ther* 1983; 63:1448–1459.

5

Determinants of Abnormal Motor Control

Pamela W. Duncan, M.A., P.T.
Mary Beth Badke, M.S., P.T.

The movement disorders of stroke have been described as being stereotypic, uncoordinated, inflexible, and nonfunctional. These descriptors have been helpful in qualitative analysis of movement dysfunction. They do not, however, help identify the specific determinants of abnormal motor control. In the past, clinicians have assumed that spasticity is the primary cause of poor volitional movement and abnormal postural control. Close clinical assessment and recent research, however, have challenged this assumption and suggested that spasticity is only one symptom of CNS damage and not necessarily the one that causes the greatest disability. Individual stroke patients exhibit varying mixtures and intensities of deficits in the components (perception-cognition, range of motion, strength, sensation, tone, synergies, and adaptability) of movement (Fig 5–1). We do assess these components when we evaluate stroke patients, some in detail and systematically, and others only grossly and unsystematically. We have failed, however, to critically analyze their interrelations and their specific contributions to movement dysfunction. Hence, our assessment of movement disorders in stroke has been unorganized and ill-defined.

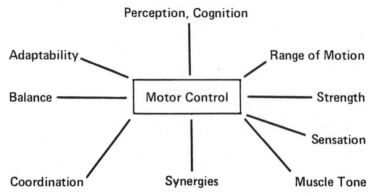

FIG 5–1.
Prerequisites for normal movement.

In order to help us more clearly delineate the specific determinants of movement dysfunction and their interrelations in stroke, we have developed a hierarchically organized model for analyzing the deficiencies in the components of motor control following stroke. The second purpose of this model is to present a unified approach to realistic program planning and selection of treatment strategies for stroke rehabilitation. In current stroke rehabilitation, we have identified components of movement dysfunction. We have not, however, interrelated the individual deficiencies.

In establishing our conceptual model (Fig 5–2), we have borrowed and expanded an analogy used by Gelfand: "Movement is a language."[17] The first prerequisite for language is the ability to perceive, think, and to understand a concept. In motor control, one must get the idea of the movement, selectively attend to the environmental conditions, and develop a motor plan. Once the movement concept is understood, the motor task is planned, and the letters (the elemental units of the language) are present, words can be developed. The letters of the movement language are range of motion, strength, muscle tone, and sensation. Adequate range of motion provides many degrees of freedom for movement, and the appropriate muscle forces acting upon the levers of the skeleton produce the movement. Normal muscle tone and sensation play important roles in increasing the efficiency and accuracy of motor performance. Every movement is constructed from the contraction of a few muscles, but there are thousands of combinations of contractions of these muscles to produce unique and purposeful movements. These functionally related patterns of muscle contractions are called synergies. Some of the muscles in synergies are primary movers (carrying the limb to the determined target or position), while other muscles are stabilizers (providing balance and equilibrium). A fundamental characteristic of synergies is that stabilization of posture precedes any movement. Finally, our language is only complete if we develop a functional vocabulary. The vocabulary of the movement language includes activation of selected synergies that are characterized by adaptability, efficiency, and accuracy.

Stroke patients have "language of movement" problems. They may not have the appropriate letters, the ability to construct words, or an adequate vocabulary. Depending on the severity of the stroke, the patient may have deficiencies in any or all of these factors. It is important to recognize that the

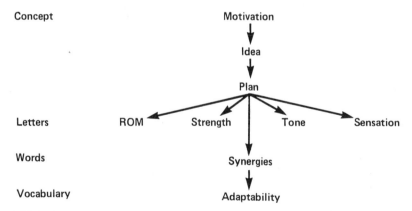

FIG 5–2.
Model for analyzing components of motor control. *ROM,* range of motion. (Data from Gelfand IM, et al: Some problems in the analysis of movements, in Gelfand IM (ed): *Models of Structural-Functional Organization of Certain Biological Systems.* Cambridge, Mass, MIT Press, 1971, pp 329–345.)

components of normal movement are hierarchically organized. If the letters are not present, the words cannot be developed; and if the words are limited, so will be the vocabulary. This hierarchical model is a tool for specifically identifying the factors that are contributing to the movement dysfunction, and it will assist us in establishing organized and realistic treatment programs.

CONCEPT

PERCEPTION AND COGNITION

In motor learning the performer must be able to selectively attend and appropriately perceive his environment. He must also be able to understand the past and relate his movement to past experience (memory). Many stroke patients have impairment in these cognitive and perceptual abilities, resulting in compromised motor performance. Several investigators have demonstrated that cognition and perception are important prognostic indicators of the functional outcomes of stroke.[1, 6, 36, 54] Spontaneous recovery of cognitive-perceptual impairments tends to be restricted by age, and the type and size of the lesion. Some currently available studies suggest that recovery of memory and perceptual deficits may be facilitated by using cognitive retraining, and several different strategies have been developed.[20, 35, 38, 77] Without recovery of cognitive function, motor relearning will be extremely limited.

Apraxia is another example of cortical brain dysfunction that contributes to the motor deficits of stroke. Apraxia, which is more frequently observed in right hemisphere damage, is a motor disorder that occurs independently of any impairment in the mechanisms of motor execution or sensory systems. It is a disorder of voluntary movement resulting from a disturbance in the ability to motor plan (ideational apraxia), or the incapacity to appropriately sequence motor patterns (idiokinetic apraxia), or the dissolution of motor patterns (motor apraxia).[52] Little research has considered the spontaneous recovery of apraxia. Hier et al.[21] report from their analysis of recovery of a few types of apraxia (in an older group of patients) that recovery is independent of sex and age. Recovery is better for patients with small lesions and in those patients whose lesions are due to hemorrhage rather than infarction.

Cognitive and perceptual functions are primary prerequisites for motor control and motor learning. Clinicians must consider the patient's cognitive and perceptual status when treating stroke. Overstressing the patient's cognitive abilities in rehabilitation can increase the effort of movement and impair motor performance. Understanding the patient's cognitive and perceptual limitations will improve the clinician's ability to realistically plan rehabilitation programs and select intervention strategies.

LETTERS

RANGE OF MOTION

The paralysis and immobilization associated with stroke predisposes most patients to contractures and subsequent loss of range of motion. Immobilization of a joint decreases the flexibility of connective tissue. Woo et al.[80] reported that following 8 weeks of joint immobilization, tissue resistance to stretch increased six times, and 50% of the increased resistance to stretch was within the muscle and skin. The increased tissue resistance is due to chemical changes and increased density of the connective tissue. A second effect of immobilization and subsequent contractures is accelerated disuse atrophy. Animal experiments have demonstrated that muscles immobilized in shortened positions have a 40% decrease in sarcomere number, a relative increase in connective tissue, and decreased rate of protein synthesis.[9, 18, 19, 63] Some researchers have attributed these physiologic changes to the loss of the trophic influence of stretch on muscle tissue. The functional effects of these changes are increased atrophy and decreased muscular force production.

A fundamental problem caused by contractures is an alteration of normal biomechanical alignment.[58] An altered biomechanical alignment will contribute to excessive effort in movement, altered movement synergies, and increased tone, as well as producing gait deviations and faulty posture.

In summary, range of motion is a key letter in the movement language, because it provides functional excursions of muscle, allows normal biomechanical alignment, and may minimize disuse atrophy.

SENSATION

Many stroke patients have major somatosensory and kinesthetic deficits. Their hemisensory losses contribute to abnormal motor control and hinder motor learning. Several research studies have demonstrated that unilateral deafferentation can result in disuse of the involved limb, unless forced training follows the sensory loss[27, 28, 34, 47, 48, 59]; yet other research studies have minimized the effect of sensory loss on residual movements in bilaterally deafferented animals.[67–73] However, closer analysis of the deafferentation studies reveal that deafferentation does cause major motor impairments. Movements are slow, clumsy, less precise, and less accurate; and deafferented animals require more time to learn new motor skills than do sensory-intact animals. In the absence of sensation, simple uniarthrodial movements and gross repetitive motor skills show minimal deficits, whereas complex and multiarthrodial movements demonstrate greater deficits.[29] In addition, monkeys that were studied following complete hemideafferentation were more incapacitated than those who had unilateral single-extremity deafferentation.[28]

In one reported case of impaired sensation from a cortical lesion in a human subject, the sensory deficits produced motor impairments in voluntary movement. The patient's motor control was slowed and limited to simple monoarticular movements that did not require coordination between fingers. The subject had difficulty maintaining a given level of muscle contraction, and there was excessive cocontraction of agonistic and antagonistic muscles.[25]

Consequently, from the previous research studies and clinical report, we may conclude that some of the frequently seen motor control problems in stroke, such as cocontraction, slow initiation of movement, inability to sustain a muscle contraction, slow velocity of movement, inability to combine limb synergies, and decreased accuracy and efficiency, may be attributed to sensory impairment as well as to involvement of the motor system itself.

The degree of sensory impairment in acute stroke may be one of the predictors for motor recovery. Leo and Soderberg[37] reported that patients with proprioceptive deficits have difficulty combining limb synergies. Kusoffsky et al.[31] found a good correlation between somatosensory function as graded by somatosensory-evoked potentials and the degree of motor recovery in stroke. This correlation was stronger for recovery of motor function in the upper extremity than the lower extremity, which may be indicative of a greater importance of sensory inputs for coordination of arm and hand movements than for leg movements.

In summary, two-way communication between the sensory and motor apparatus is a fundamental prerequisite for accuracy and efficiency in movement. Without this sensorimotor link, motor learning during stroke rehabilitation will be severely impaired.

STRENGTH

Muscular strength is defined as "the capacity of a muscle to produce the tension necessary for maintaining posture, initiating movement, or controlling movement during conditions of loading on the musculoskeletal system."[62] In stroke patients, weakness or paresis is a primary motor deficit. Patients are unable to generate normal muscle tension, and they often experience a tremendous sense of effort when they produce minimal muscular force. Understanding the role of strength limitation on movement dysfunction in stroke, therefore, is an important goal for clinicians. In the past, strength deficits have been attributed to spasticity of antagonistic muscle groups. More recently, however, researchers have demonstrated that many factors appear to contribute to the weakness of stroke.

The amount of muscle force produced by a muscle contraction is dependent upon (1) the number of motor units recruited, (2) the type of motor units recruited, and (3) the motor unit discharge frequency. Recent research has demonstrated that in patients with hemiplegia, one or all of these mechanisms may be affected. McComas et al.[41] reported that there is a reduction in the number of functioning motor units in a small foot muscle in hemiplegic subjects. This reduction was interpreted to be the result of transsynaptic alterations of spinal motor neurons. Second, structural and physiologic alterations of muscle fibers and neuromuscular junctions following upper motor neuron lesions have been reported. Atrophy of muscles in hemiplegic subjects have been recognized by clinicians for many years, and recent histochemical studies by Edstrom[13] demonstrated a decrease in the number of muscle fibers, and a selective atrophy of fast-twitch fibers. The degree of fast-twitch fiber atrophy was directly related to the degree of paresis. In another study, Edstrom et al.[14] reported that the degree of fast-fiber atrophy was directly related to the degree of spasticity. Subjects with marked spasticity had selective atrophy of fast-twitch fibers, while those with minimal spasticity had atrophy of both slow and fast. Chokroverty et al.[12] found atrophy of both fast- and slow-twitch muscle fibers, but with a predominance of fast-twitch atrophy. Sjostrom et al.[61] reported fiber dedifferentiation and the transformation from slow- to fast-muscle fiber predominance in both legs of hemiplegic subjects. Mayer and Young[40] reported a differential effect on fast- and slow-twitch units in the first dorsal interosseus muscle of hemiplegic subjects. In acute flaccid hemiplegia the contraction time of fast units was increased without changes in twitch tension. In long-term hemiplegia, the twitch tension of slow units became greater. These changes were attributed to alterations in motor unit activity and excitability secondary to hemiplegia.[40] A third factor that may result in weakness of hemiplegic subjects is the abnormal central control of motor neuron firing. Several investigators have reported an abnormal and reduced firing rate of motor neurons in patients with upper motor neuron lesions. Specifically, Rosenfalck and Andreassen[56] reported that patients with spastic hemiparesis are unable to generate normal force, partly because motor units exhibit a reduced firing rate at a high level of contraction and lack the rapid regulation of firing rate that is characteristic of normal muscle contraction.

Tang and Rymer[64] examined the relation between electromyography (EMG) and isometric force generated by the normal and paretic elbow flexors of 14 hemiparetic subjects. In almost half of the subjects, the amount of EMG produced per unit of force was significantly increased in the paretic elbow flexors (Fig 5–3). Simultaneous EMG recordings from the triceps did not reveal excessive cocontraction. Tang and Rymer concluded that

> *reductions in force output for each motor unit would mean that many more motor units would have to be activated if the muscle were to reach some required level of force. This situation could give rise to weakness when all readily accessible motor units are recruited, and to an increased effort at lower levels of activation, since a stronger central command would be required to generate a given level of force.*[64]

Several authors who have written about their own strokes describe precisely this sense of effort during volitional movement.[10, 26]

Whitley, et al.[79] analyzed patterns of EMG activity in the upper extremity of 14 chronic hemiplegic patients. During wrist movements, EMG activity was recorded from wrist flexors and extensors, biceps, triceps, and pectoralis major and trapezius muscles. They concluded that the primary deficit in wrist

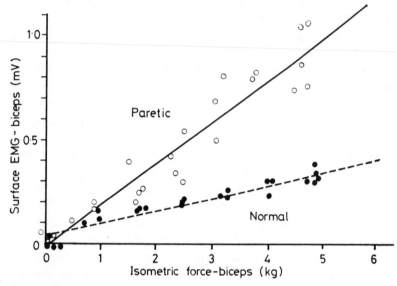

FIG 5–3.
Mean force-EMG data and corresponding regression lines from biceps-brachialis muscle groups of 14 stroke subjects. Note that the slope derived for the *paretic* limb is greater than that of the *normal* limb. (From Tang A, Rymer WZ: Abnormal force-EMG relations in paretic limbs of hemiparetic human subjects. *J Neurol Neurosurg Psychiatry* 1981; 44:690–698. Used by permission.)

movement is not due to abnormal cocontraction of antagonistic muscle groups or hyperreflexia. Instead, they noted paucity of motor unit activity and abnormal synergistic patterns.[79]

In summary, the paresis of hemiplegia is not due solely to an overactive antagonistic muscle, but may be caused by alterations in motor unit discharge patterns and reduced firing rate caused by damage to supraspinal descending systems. Actual changes in muscle fibers that are characteristic of stroke patients further limit the muscle's ability to produce force. The ability to produce an efficient muscle contraction is the basic letter of any movement. If the muscles cannot efficiently contract, postural and movement synergies will not develop, effort of movement will be excessive, and functional performance will be very limited.

MUSCLE TONE

Muscle tone is a term used to describe the tension attained at any moment between the origin and the insertion of a muscle. The tension is determined partly by mechanical factors (connective tissue and viscoelastic properties of muscles) and the degree of motor unit activity.[81] Tone is usually assessed clinically by moving an extremity alternately while the patient relaxes. The resistance to passive movement is supposed to reflect the sensitivity of the stretch reflex mechanism.

Spasticity is not a clearly defined term. Many times the word spasticity simply refers to an increased resistance to passive stretch (hypertonicity). Landau,[33] however, presented at least six different definitions of spasticity, while Wyn Jones and Mulley[83] discussed three viewpoints of spasticity: clinical, physical therapy, and neurophysiologic. In the current language of stroke rehabilitation, the term *spasticity* is used to signify any of the following phenomena: (1) hyperactive stretch reflex, (2) increased resistance to passive movement, (3) posturing of the upper extremity in flexion and the lower extremity in extension, (4) excessive cocontraction of antagonistic muscles, and (5) stereotypic movement synergies. Spasticity is therefore not one particular disorder of motor control, but usually results from a variety of neurophysiologic causes. In an effort to help us solve this clinical dilemma, Lance[32] defines spasticity in more restrictive terms: "Spasticity is a velocity-dependent increase in the tonic stretch reflex with exaggerated tendon jerks resulting from hyperexcitability of the stretch reflex as one component of the upper motor neuron syndrome."

Stroke patients often present with abnormal tone. Initially, the patient is hypotonic (flaccid) and offers little resistance to passive movement. As recovery progresses, the tone increases abnormally. The relation of tone to abnormal movement is not completely understood. Clinicians have reported that "spasticity must be held responsible for much of a patient's motor deficits" and "weakness of muscles may not be real but relative to the opposition of the spastic antagonist. If the latter of spasticity is reduced, this 'weak' muscle may show normal power."[8] Hughlings Jackson,[76] however, categorized the dysfunction of neurologic lesions into two distinct sets of symptoms, negative and positive. Negative symptoms were defined as deficits of normal behavior and positive symptoms as a release phenomenon. In stroke, the inability to move is an example of a negative symptom, while spasticity is an example of a positive symptom. Hughlings Jackson concluded that the positive and negative symptoms were two separate entities that may be related, but do not have a cause-effect relationship. Landau[33] suggested that the negative symptoms (weakness and inability to move) are the most disabling to the stroke patient, while the development of spasticity may assist function. For example, quadriceps spasticity stiffens the knee for functional weight bearing.

The pathophysiology of the spasticity is as controversial as the clinical definition of spasticity. For many years it has been thought that spasticity is caused by hyperactivity of the stretch reflex secondary to excessive gamma motor neuron activity. More recently many researchers are beginning to challenge this theory. Sahrmann and Norton's[57] assessment of EMG activity of elbow flexors and extensors in 16 patients with upper motoneuron lesions during repetitive movement revealed that the motor deficits were due to limited and prolonged recruitment of the agonist contraction and delayed cessation of the contraction at the end of movement. The probable explanation for this finding is not the hypersensitivity of the stretch reflex, but rather abnormal supraspinal regulation of the motor neuron pool. McLellan[42] compared the EMG activity of the quadriceps and hamstrings of 11 spastic patients during passive and active movements. He demonstrated the response of a spastic muscle to stretch is not the same during passive motion as during active movement. He concluded that the emphasis on the hypersensitivity of the stretch reflex as a cause of motor disorders should be reexamined. Miller and Hammond[46] demonstrated that motor control disturbances in the upper extremity of stroke patients are probably due to disorders of reciprocal inhibition between antagonistic muscle groups, thereby increasing resistance to voluntary movement. Yanagisawa et al.[84] also noted disorders in reciprocal inhibition in the lower extremity of hemiparetic patients. The picture that emerges from this experimental data is that the hypertonicity or spasticity we observe in stroke is not simply due to the hyperactive stretch reflex, but rather due to abnormal programming and regulation of the motor neuron pool for selective and coordinated movement.

Clinicians should realize that in stroke rehabilitation it is more appropriate to concentrate upon reestablishing normal active motor control rather than reducing the hypersensitivity of the stretch reflex in response to passive movement. Coordination and regulation of the motor neuron pool for reciprocal movements is a necessary letter for efficiency and accuracy in motor control.

WORDS

SYNERGIES

Normal movement does not consist of isolated muscle actions that are volitionally controlled but rather consists of functionally related patterns of muscle contractions called synergies. In synergies the muscle contractions are varied in sequence to produce effective and efficient movements which are adaptable to the changing circumstances of movement execution. Synergies include not only the muscle activity in the extremities which produce the movement, but also muscle activity which stabilizes the body during movement. Over 100 years ago Ferrier suggested that movements were the result of large integrated actions of the nervous system. He wrote "every form of active muscular exertion necessitates the simultaneous cooperation of an immense assemblage of synergic movements throughout the body to secure steadiness and maintain equilibrium."[16] A century later, Bernstein also recognized the importance of viewing movements as synergistically organized. Bernstein said that movements were not to be viewed as "chains of details but as structures, which are differentiated into details: they are structurally whole." He argued that synergies are essential because the brain can not individually control the many muscle groups and mechanical couplings that occur during movement. Functional synergies simplify the control of movement for the CNS.[7]

A characteristic of synergies is that contraction of muscles is spatially and temporally sequenced, with muscles contracting in bursts of activity rather than in synchronized, sustained contraction.[23] Indeed, coordinated movement is characterized by appropriate timing and sequence of muscle activation.

Of interest in the discussion of synergies is the description of motor behaviors in developmental neurology. For many years our analysis of movement and movement deficits has been restricted by the Sherringtonian philosophy, which is the reflexology point of view.[59] Many of our primary movements are considered reflexes (tonic neck reflex, optical righting reflex, labyrinthine reflexes, etc.). Reflexologists suggest that reflexes produce postural attitudes and that complex behaviors are a concoction of reflexes.[39] Review of neuroembryologic studies of motor behavior, however, challenges the reflexology point of view. As early as 1885, Preyer[55] observed spontaneous activity in the chick embryo several days before sensory stimulation-evoked reflexes. The presence of prereflexogenic periods of mobility may support the point of view that many of our prenatal movements are endogenously generated and are the precursors of a more complex motor pattern. Milani Comparetti[44] reports, on the basis of human fetal movement observations, that many of our "primitive movements or reflexes are primary motor programs: genetic modules which are genetic endowments of the species and are available for motor programming."[45] Patterns of gross flexion and extension were the first primary motor programs identified by Milani Comparetti. These normal fetal movements are disorganized, random, and jerky in appearance. Milani Comparetti parallels the stereotypic movements observed in persons with CNS damage with these primary motor programs. The problem in stroke patients is that the stereotypic movements are not modified and expanded upon like the primary motor programs are in normal motor development. Milani Comparetti concludes, therefore, that "abnormality is not the acquisition of abnormal movements but is the loss of normal movement."[43-45]

In contrast to the variety and flexibility observed in normal movement, stroke patients' movements are inflexible and non-selective. The stereotypic movement patterns in hemiplegia occur in predictable patterns that are not adapted to the change in environmental demands of the movement. Brunnstrom[11] described these patterns in detail and promoted keen observation of them for assessment of motor function in stroke patients (Table 5–1).[11]

The relationship of spasticity to the stereotypic movement synergies observed in stroke has been ill-defined. Clinically we have observed that the stereotypic synergies of stroke often wax and wane together with the degree of spasticity (flaccid

TABLE 5–1.
Stereotypic Movement Synergies of Stroke*

FLEXOR SYNERGY	EXTENSOR SYNERGY
UPPER EXTREMITY	
Elbow flexion	Elbow extension
Forearm supination	Forearm pronation
External rotation of shoulder	Internal rotation of shoulder
Abduction of shoulder	Adduction of shoulder
Retraction/elevation of shoulder girdle	Protraction of shoulder girdle
LOWER EXTREMITY	
Toe dorsiflexion	Toe plantarflexion
Dorsiflexion and inversion of ankle	Ankle plantarflexion and inversion
Knee flexion	Knee extension
Hip flexion	Hip extension
Hip abduction and external rotation	Hip adduction and internal rotation

*Adapted from Brunnstrom S: *Movement Therapy in Hemiplegia.* New York, Harper & Row, 1970, pp 8–10.

tone, no synergistic movement; spastic tone, stereotypic syner-gies; normal tone, selective control).[8, 11] However, the rela-tionship between spasticity and selective control should not be considered a cause-and-effect relation. Our therapeutic in-terventions that reduce abnormal muscle tone do not neces-sarily increase volitional selective motor control.[43–45] For ex-ample, a common clinical problem in stroke is a flexed wrist with fisted hand. Therapists are usually able to reduce the flexor tone with slow stroking and slow passive manipulation or rotation, and yet the patient is still unable to extend the wrist and hand volitionally in a normal movement pattern. Both spastic and limited movement patterns are signs of CNS dysfunction caused by pathologic mechanisms, but one sign of CNS dysfunction does not necessarily cause another sign of CNS dysfunction.[75] In summary, stereotypic synergies ob-served in stroke and spasticity are related but independent phenomena.

The development of the language of movement depends upon a spatial-temporal configuration of muscle activity to pro-duce movement patterns. A primary goal of stroke rehabilita-tion is to increase the variety of synergies by breaking down the stereotypic movements into smaller components of move-ment, recombining these components into an increased num-ber of movement options, and, finally, expanding upon these new movement patterns and increasing their adaptability.

Postural adjustments in standing are a functional example of a synergy. Nashner and Horak[24, 49–51] have recently developed a model for analyzing these adjustments. They have shown that, in normal subjects, the postural responses to perturbation while standing on a flat movable platform are characterized by (1) fixed patterns of muscle activity that are specific for the direction of displacement, (2) fixed spatial and temporal char-acteristics of muscle contractions, and (3) a sequence of mus-cle activity beginning distally and moving proximally. The components of a normal postural adjustment include range of motion, biomechanical alignment, muscular strength, coordi-nation, and sensory organization. The somatosensory and vi-sual inputs are particularly important for maintaining balance, and the vestibular system appears to play a role in the resolution of sensory conflict.

Stroke patients frequently present with deficits in postural adaptations. Badke and Duncan's[3] analysis of the postural adjustments of ten stroke patients revealed that some of the patients had inconsistent patterns of muscular activity, excessive muscular cocontraction, longer and more varied response latencies, and distorted sequences of muscular activation. The pathophysiology underlying these abnormal postural adjustments in stroke patients is not clear in the current research. Problems with descending commands, which may influence propriospinal circuits and alterations in long-loop reflex mechanisms, may contribute to the postural dysfunction. Poor synergistic organization of the automatic movement patterns at the higher levels also may be a factor. Finally, abnormal sensory inputs or altered sensory integration at all levels may hinder normal postural adaptations. Biomechanical factors such as velocity of movement, and initial standing posture appear to affect postural response strategies used, and must be considered when evaluating the stroke patient.[4,5]

VOCABULARY

ADAPTABILITY

Adaptability is the flexibility in the CNS that allows it to produce relevant and effective voluntary or automatic movements in a variety of environmental contexts or situational demands. The degrees of freedom for functional movements are maximized, allowing the individual to appropriately interact with his environment. Factors that the CNS must assess prior to and during movement to ensure the adaptability of the response are (a) body position, (b) amplitude of movement, (c) force requirements, (d) posture requirements, (e) speed requirements, (f) accuracy requirements, (g) sensory and environmental conditions, and (h) the current status of the muscle activity in the body.

In order for the CNS to assess necessary movement variables and display adaptability, the letters (range of motion, tone, strength, sensation) and the words (synergies) must be available. The CNS must have the capability to modify these motor programs; to assess the environmental context, movement requirements, and body position; and to make predictions. Finally, one must have the cognitive and perceptual capabilities for motor planning. Each movement is unique and requires alterations of the motor strategies available in the CNS. Sensorimotor communication before, during, and at the termination of movement is important for this adaptability.

In stroke patients the movement response to various demands is often rigid and inflexible, accentuating their motor dysfunction. This dysfunction may be evident by (1) increased tone, (2) loss of selectivity of movement, (3) lack of automatic movements, (4) difficulty in moving into antigravity positions, (5) inability to carry volitional movements over into the functional tasks, (6) the inability to control finely graded movement, and (7) an inability to move at different velocities.

Clinically, adaptability of motor responses in stroke patients can be evaluated by assessing movement responses in a variety of positions (supine, sitting, standing, and walking) and situations (voluntary, functional, automatic, stress and nonstress, a variety of movement amplitudes, variety of force requirements, and a variety of speed requirements). The patient's ability to coordinate muscular activity in a variety of conditions and under a number of different circumstances is a sign of a more advanced motor control and good communication between the CNS and the environment.

SUMMARY

To realistically plan treatment programs and select intervention strategies, we need to analyze more carefully the determinants of movement dysfunction and their interrelations. The model presented in this chapter for analyzing the components of motor control should be a useful problem-solving tool for most clinicians. Using this model, the clinician will (1) identify the motor deficits, (2) determine which components of motor control are abnormal, and (3) decide which abnormal components are the primary cause of the deficit.

REFERENCES

1. Adams GF: *Cerebrovascular Disability and the Ageing Brain.* Edinburgh and London, Churchill Livingstone, 1974.
2. Andreassen S: Single motor unit recording, in Feldman RG, Young RR, Koella WP (eds): *Spasticity: Disordered Motor Control.* Chicago, Year Book Medical Publishers, 1980.
3. Badke MB, Duncan PW: Patterns of rapid motor responses in normal and hemiplegic subjects during postural adjustments in standing. *Phys Ther* 1983; 63:13–20.
4. Badke MB, DiFabio RP, Duncan, PW: Laterality of rapid motor responses in hemiplegic subjects during dysequilibrium in standing. *Phys Ther* 1985; 65:715.
5. Badke MB, DiFabio RP: Effects of postural bias during support surface displacements and rapid arm movements. *Phys Ther* 1985; 65:1490–1495.
6. Ben-Yishay Y, Gerstman L, Diller L, et al: Prediction of the rehabilitation outcomes from psychometric parameters in left hemiplegics. *J Consult Clin Psychol* 1970; 34:436–441.
7. Bernstein N: *The Co-ordination and Regulation of Movements.* Oxford, Pergamon Press, 1967.
8. Bobath B: *Adult Hemiplegia: Evaluation and Treatment.* London, William Heinemann, 1978.
9. Booth FW, Seider MJ: Early changes in skeletal muscle protein synthesis after limb immobilization of rats. *J Appl Physiol* 1979; 47:974–977.
10. Brodal A: Self-observations and neuro-anatomical considerations after a stroke. *Brain* 1973; 96:675–694.
11. Brunnstrom S: *Movement Therapy in Hemiplegia.* New York, Harper & Row, 1970.
12. Chokroverty S, Reyes MG, Rubino FA, et al: Hemiplegic amyotrophy. *Arch Neurol* 1976; 33:104–110.
13. Edstrom L: Selective changes in the sizes of red and white muscle fibers in upper motor lesions and parkinsonism. *J Neurol Sci* 1970; 11:537–550.

14. Edstrom L, Grimby L, Hannerz J: Correlation between recruitment order of motor units and muscle atrophy patterns of upper motor neuron lesions: Significance of spasticity. *Experientia* 1973; 29:560–561.

15. Eidelberg E, Davis F: Role of proprioceptive data in performance of a complex visuomotor tracking task. *Brain Res* 1976; 105:588–590.

16. Ferrier D: *The Functions of the Brain,* ed 2. London, Smith, Elder & Co, 1886.

17. Gelfand IM, et al: Some problems in the analysis of movements, in Gelfand IM (ed): *Models of Structural-Functional Organization of Certain Biological Systems.* Cambridge, Mass, MIT Press, 1971, pp 329–345.

18. Goldspink DF: The influence of immobilization and stretch on protein turnover of rat skeletal muscle. *J Physiol* 1977; 264:267–282.

19. Goldspink DF: The influence of activity on muscle size and protein turnover. *J Physiol* 1977; 264:283–296.

20. Harris JE: Methods of improving memory, in Wilson B, Moffat N, (eds): *Clinical Management of Memory Problems.* London, Croom Helm, 1984.

21. Hier DB, Mondlock J, Caplan LR: Recovery of behavioural abnormalities after right hemisphere stroke. *Neurology* 1983b; 33:345–350.

22. Hocherman S, Dickstein R, Pillaw F: Platform training and postural stability in hemiplegia. *Arch Phys Med Rehabil* 1984; 65:588–592.

23. Horak RB, Esselman P, Anderson ME, et al: The effects of movement velocity, mass displaced, and task certainty on associated postural adjustments made by normal and hemiplegic individuals. *J Neurol Neurosurg Psychiatry* 1984; 47:1020–1028.

24. Horak FB, Nashner LM: Two distinct strategies for stance posture control: Adaptation to altered support surface configurations. *Neurosci Res Bull* November, 1983.

25. Jeannerod M, Michel F, Prablanc C: The control of hand movements in a case of hemianaesthesia following parietal lesion. *Brain* 1984; 101:899–920.

26. Chapman RW (ed): *The Letters of Samuel Johnson.* Oxford, Clarendon Press, 1952, vol 3, pp 30, 40.

27. Knapp HD, Taub E, Berman AJ: Effect of deafferentation on a conditioned avoidance response. *Science* 1958; 128:842–843.
28. Knapp HD, Taub E, Berman AJ: Movements in monkeys with deafferented forelimbs. *Exp Neurol* 1963; 7:305–315.
29. Kots YM, Krinsky VI, Naydin VL, et al: The control of movements of the joints and kinesthetic afferentation, in Gelfand IM (ed): *Models of Structural-Functional Organization of Certain Biological Systems.* Cambridge, Mass, MIT Press, 1971, pp 373–381.
30. Kranz H: Control of motoneuron firing during maintained voluntary contractions with central lesions. *Prog Clin Neurophysiol* 1981; 9:359–367.
31. Kusoffsky A, Wadell I, Nilsson BY: The relationship between sensory impairment and motor recovery in patients with hemiplegia. *Scand J Rehabil Med* 1982; 14:27–32.
32. Lance JW: Symposium synopsis, in Feldman RG, Young RR, Koella WP (eds): *Spasticity: Disordered Motor Control.* Miami, Symposia Specialists, 1977, pp 485–494.
33. Landau WM: Spasticity: What is it? What is it not? in Feldman RG, Young RR, Koella WP (eds): *Spasticity: Disordered Motor Control.* Miami, Symposia Specialists, 1977, pp 17–24.
34. Lassek AM: Inactivation of voluntary motor function following rhizotomy. *J Neuropathol Exp Neurol* 1953; 3:83–87.
35. Leftoff S: Learning functions for unilaterally brain-damaged patients for serially and randomly ordered stimulus material: Analysis of retrieval strategies and their relationship to rehabilitation. *J Clin Neuropsychol* 1981; 3:301–314.
36. Lehmann JR, DeLateur BJ, Fowler RS, et al: Stroke rehabilitation outcome and prediction. *Arch Phys Med Rehabil* 1975b; 56:383–389.
37. Leo KC, Soderberg GC: Relationship between perception of joint position sense and limb synergies in patients with hemiplegia. *Phys Ther* 1982; 61:1433–1437.
38. Lewinsohn PM, Glasgow RE, Barrera M, et al: Assessment and treatment of patients with memory deficits: Initial studies. *JSAS* (catalogue of selected documents in psychology) 1977; 7 (3): 1–139.
39. Magnus R: Some results of studies in the physiology of posture. *Lancet* 1926; 211:531–536, 585–588.
40. Mayer RF, Young JL: The effects of hemiplegia with spasticity, in

Feldman RG, Young RR, Koella WP (eds): *Spasticity: Disordered Motor Control.* Chicago, Year Book Medical Publishers, 1980.

41. McComas AJ, Sica RE, Upton AR, et al: Functional changes in motoneurons of hemiparetic patients. *J Neurol Neurosurg Psychiatry* 1973; 36:183–193.
42. McLellan DL: Co-contraction and stretch reflex in spasticity during treatment with baclofen. *Neurol Neurosurg Psychiatry* 1977; 40:30–38.
43. Milani Comparetti A: Spasticity vs postural and motor behavior of spastics, in *Proceedings of the Fourth International Congress of Physical Medicine.* New York, Excerpta Medica, 1964.
44. Milani Comparetti A: The neurophysiologic and clinical implications of studies on fetal motor behavior. *Semin Perinatol* 1981; 5:183–189.
45. Milani Comparetti A: Fetal movements and developmental prognosis, in Slaton D (ed): *Developmental Movement in Infancy: A Symposium.* Chapel Hill, University of North Carolina, 1981.
46. Miller S, Hammond GR: Neural control of arm movement in patients following stroke, in Van Hof MW, Mohn G (ed): *Functional Recovery from Brain Damage.* Amsterdam, Elsevier/New Holland, 1981, pp 259–274.
47. Mott FW, Sherrington CS: Experiments upon the influence of sensory nerves upon movement and nutrition of the limbs. *Proc R Soc Lond* 1985; 57:481–488.
48. Munk H: *Ueber die Functionen von Hirn und Ruckenmark.* Berlin, Hirshwald, 1909, pp 247–285.
49. Nashner LM: Adapting reflexes controlling the human posture. *Exp Brain Res* 1976; 26:59–72.
50. Nashner LM: Fixed patterns of rapid postural responses among leg muscles during stance. *Exp Brain Res* 1977; 30:13–24.
51. Nashner LM: The organization of rapid postural adjustments of standing humans: An experimental conceptual model, in Talbott, RE, Humphey DR (eds): *Posture and Movement.* New York, Raven Press, 1979, pp 243–257.
52. Palliard J: The patterning of skilled movements, in Field J (ed): *Handbook of Physiology: Neurophysiology III.* Washington, DC, American Physiological Society, 1960.
53. Petajan JH: Motor unit control in spasticity, in Feldman RG, Young RR, Koella WP (eds): *Spasticity: Disordered Motor Control.* Chicago, Year Book Medical Publishers, 1980.

54. Prescott RJ, Garraway WM, Akhtar AJ: Predicting functional outcome following acute stroke using a standard clinical examination. *Stroke* 1982; 13:641–647.
55. Preyer W: *Specielle physiologie des embryo.* Leipzig, Germany, Grieben, 1885.
56. Rosenfalck A, Andreassen S: Impaired regulation of force and firing pattern of single motor units in patients with spasticity. *Neurol Neurosurg Psychiatry* 1980; 43:907–916.
57. Sahrmann SA, Norton BS: The relationship of voluntary movement to spasticity in the upper motoneuron syndrome. *Ann Neurol* 1977; 2:460–465.
58. Sharpless JW: Contractures: Pathophysiology, prevention and treatment, in Sharpless JW: *A Problem-Oriented Approach to Stroke Rehabilitation.* Springfield, Ill, Charles C Thomas, Publisher, 1982, pp 62–66.
59. Sherrington CS: *The Integrated Action of the Nervous System.* London, Constable, 1906.
60. Sica R, Sanz O: An electrophysiological study of the functional changes in the spinal motoneurons of hemiparetic patients. *Electromyogr Clin Neurophysiol* 1976; 16:419–431.
61. Sjostrom R, Fugl-Meyer AR, Nordin G, et al: Post-stroke hemiplegia: Crural muscle strength and structure. *Scand J Rehabil Med* 1980; suppl 7, pp 53–67.
62. Smidt GL, Rogers MW: Factors contributing to the regulation and clinical assessment of muscular strength. *Phys Ther* 1982; 62:1283–1290.
63. Tabary JC, Tabary C, Tardieu G, et al: Physiological and structural changes in the cat's soleus muscle due to immobilization at different lengths by plaster casts. *J Physiol* 1972; 224:231–244.
64. Tang A, Rymer WZ: Abnormal force-EMG relations in paretic limbs of hemiparetic human subjects. *Neurol Neurosurg Psychiatry* 1981; 44:690–698.
65. Taub E: Somatosensory deafferentation research with monkeys: Implications for rehabilitation medicine, in Ince LP (ed): *Behavior Psychology in Rehabilitation Medicine.* Baltimore, Williams & Wilkins Co, 1980.
66. Taub E, Barro G, Parker B, et al: Utility of a limb following unilateral deafferentation in monkeys, paper read at Neuroscience Society Meeting, Houston, October 1972.
67. Taub E, Berman AJ: Avoidance conditioning in the absence of

relevant proprioceptive and exteroceptive feedback. *J Comp Physiol Psychol* 1963; 56:1012–1016.

68. Taub E, Bacon R, Berman AJ: The acquisition of a trace-conditioned avoidance response after deafferentation of the responding limb. *J Comp Physiol Psychol* 1965; 58:275–279.

69. Taub E, Berman AJ: Movement and learning in the absence of sensory feedback, in Freeman SJ (ed): *The Neuropsychology of Spatially Oriented Behavior.* Homewood, Ill, Dorsey Press, 1968.

70. Taub E, Teodoru D, Ellman SJ, et al: Deafferentation in monkeys: Extinction of avoidance responses, discrimination and discrimination reversal. *Psychonom Sci* 1966; 4:323–324.

71. Taub E, Ellman SJ, Berman AJ: Deafferentation in monkeys: Effect on conditioned grasp response. *Science* 1966; 151:593–594.

72. Taub E, Goldberg IA, Taub PB: Deafferentation in monkeys: Pointing at a target without visual feedback. *Exp Neurol* 1975; 46:178–186.

73. Taub E, Schlossberg S, Teodoru D, et al: Regulation of force output with an unseen limb in deafferented monkeys (unpublished).

74. Twitchell TE: Sensory factors in purposive movement. *J Neurophysiol* 1954; 17:239–254.

75. VanSant A: Designing a definitive clinical study of spasticity. *Neurol Rep* 1985; 9:17–19.

76. Walshe F: Contributions of John Hughlings Jackson to neurology: A brief introduction to his teaching. *Arch Neurol* 1961; 5:119–131.

77. Weinberg J, Diller L, Gordon WA, et al: Training sensory awareness and spatial organization in people with right brain damage. *Arch Phys Med Rehabil* 1979; 60:491–496.

78. Weinberg J, Piasetsky E, Diller L, et al: Treatment perceptual organization deficits in non-neglecting right brain damaged stroke patients. *J Clin Neuro Psychol* 1982; 4:59–76.

79. Whitley DA, Sahrmann SA, Norton BJ: Patterns of muscle activity in the hemiplegic upper extremity. *Phys Ther* 1982; 62:641.

80. Woo SLV, Matthews JV, Akerson WH, et al: Connective tissue response to immobility. *Arthritis Rheum* 1975; 18:257–264.

81. Wyke B: Neurological mechanisms in spasticity. *Physiotherapy* 1976; 62:316–319.

82. Wylie RM: Deafferentation interferes with avoidance of muscle

fatigue during performance of a repetitive motor task, *Fed Proc* 1978, vol 37.

83. Wyn Jones E, Mulley GP: The measurement of spasticity, in Rose FC (ed): *Advances in Stroke Therapy.* New York, Raven Press, 1982, pp 187–195.
84. Yanagisawa N, Tanka R, Ito Z: Reciprocal Ia inhibition in spastic hemiplegia of man. *Brain* 1976; 96:555–574.
85. Young JL, Mayer RF: Mechanical properties of single motor units in short-term hemiplegia. *Neurology* 1979; 29:609.
86. Young RR, Shahani BT: A clinical neurophysiological analysis of single motor unit discharge patterns in spasticity, in Feldman RG, Young RR, Koella WP (eds): *Spasticity: Disordered Motor Control.* Chicago, Year Book Medical Publishers, 1980.

6

Therapeutic Strategies for Rehabilitation of Motor Deficits

Pamela W. Duncan, M.A., P.T.
Mary Beth Badke, M.S., P.T.

GOAL OF PHYSICAL THERAPY

The goal of physical therapy in stroke rehabilitation is to teach the patient to develop strategies for movement that are functional, responsive to environmental stresses, and adaptable to activities of daily living. The specific purpose of physical therapy is to maximize motor performance and minimize functional deficits within the constraints of the neurologic damage. The benefits of physical therapy may be maximized by early intervention and well-planned treatment programs. The following guidelines are critical if treatment is to produce any long-term results.

1. Utilize an analytical approach:
   a. Analyze what movement strategies, postural responses, and feedback are necessary to accomplish a movement.
   b. Decide if the patient has the prerequisites for movement.
   c. Outline the missing components for normal movement and develop the missing components using a

161

treatment strategy based on the hierarchical model presented in chapter 5.

2. Stress active performance by the patient. The environment should be appropriate for the patient's cooperation and set up in ways to challenge different aspects of an individual's capacity.[16] The training must be an active learning process in which the patient develops control of the movement.[8] The critical feature is not how can we stimulate or facilitate movement, but that the patient actively participates in the movement.

3. Exercise in the context of functional activities. Exercises that incorporate functional activities should be emphasized, because they provide the patient with meaningful goal-directed actions. Secondly, it will help facilitate the transfer of motor learning to activities of daily living.

4. Include sufficient practice under a variety of environmental conditions. Bernstein's[8] model of motor skill acquisition emphasizes that practice is a process of finding new solutions to a motor problem rather than the constant repetition of one fixed routine. This model has major implications for stroke rehabilitation, because it suggests that we should not simply repeat the same exercise routines to develop a motor skill, but rather try to increase the patient's ability to select the appropriate movement pattern in a variety of activities.

REALISTIC PROGRAM PLANNING

The predisposing factors associated with a positive or negative outcome following stroke have not been well established. Our clinical judgments, however, indicate that severe cognitive-perceptual deficits, apraxias, sensory loss, and medical complications have a negative effect on outcome. The initial severity of the patient's sensory and motor deficits may also be a predictor of outcome. A patient who presents early with low tone and isolated (even though they may be very weak) movements will recover well; yet a patient who develops moderate-to-severe hypertonicity quickly and whose movement patterns are limited to stereotypic synergies will not usually experience significant improvement in motor coordination and skill.

Optimal goals for intervention may be established by determining if the purpose of physical therapy is to (1) normalize movement and functional skills; (2) significantly improve motor function and functional skills, even though normalcy of motor control is not realistic or; (3) focus on compensatory methods to achieve functional goals while not expecting any significant change in sensorimotor status. Patients must be able to develop sensorimotor prerequisites and must be able to learn to reorganize and interpret distorted sensory input from their own internal feedback system.[3, 4] If a client is unable to learn this, it will be impossible to wean him from artificial stimulation. While performing certain tasks may be improved by using an artifical source of feedback, the patient must be able to eventually do them without the external feedback and therapist intervention. If the patient is unable to learn to utilize the sensory signals provided by his own internal feedback loops, then it is unrealistic to expect return of normal motor function.

To select unrealistic goals and continue fruitless interventions are costly and frustrating for both therapist and patient. The patient quickly loses motivation, and therapists develop "burnout."

DIAGNOSIS OF MOVEMENT DISORDER

In order to effectively treat the motor deficits of stroke, we need to be able to identify the specific determinants of the motor disorder; in other words, diagnose the movement disorder. When a physician treats heart disease, he does not treat all patients alike, but rather establishes the cause (congestive heart failure, myocardial infarction, arrhythmia) of the abnormality. Likewise, therapists should not treat all stroke patients alike. There is a great deal of interindividual variation in the motor disorders. The success of our intervention depends on our ability to clinically assess the specific causative factor of motor deficits. Diagnosing the movement disorders can be divided into six steps: observe, assess, evaluate, select intervention strategies, treat, and reevaluate (Table 6–1). Once the specific causes of the movement disorders are identified and the patient's health, age, motivation, and family support are considered, the successful clinician will establish the optimal goals for therapy. Based on these established goals, appropriate treatment strategies can be selected.

STRATEGIES FOR INTERVENTION

The objectives for treatment procedures are based on the hierarchical model presented in chapter 5 and are designed to

TABLE 6–1.
Diagnosis of the Movement Disorder

I. Observe motor deficit: inability to weight shift on involved extremity
II. Assess factors that could cause the motor deficit
    1. Perception—the patient's perception of vertical is distorted
    2. Range of motion—the patient lacks sufficient hip, knee, or ankle range of motion to provide adequate biomechanical alignment for weight shift.
    3. Tone—the patient has excessive and prolonged muscle activity in certain muscle groups
    4. Weakness—the patient cannot generate appropriate muscle force to maintain body weight or adjust to postural displacements
    5. Sensory—the patient has inadequate sensory integration to provide feedback about foot placement and weight shift
    6. Synergistic organization—the patient's movement is restricted to the stereotypic flexion and extension synergies of stroke that do not provide selective and efficient use of flexor and extensor muscle groups for postural adaptations and movements
    7. Coordination—the patient has deficits in timing and reciprocation of muscle activity
    8. Adaptability—as the speed and force requirements vary, environmental conditions change and the volitional control of the movement is reduced, the patient cannot quickly and efficiently respond to postural displacements
III. Evaluate: decide which of these factors are contributing to the patient's motor deficits
IV. Select intervention strategies
V. Treat
VI. Reevaluate—is there an improvement in functional movement patterns?

---

help the patient relearn movement patterns and postural control. The objectives are as follows:

1. Provide an environment and a variety of activities that are conducive to motor relearning.
2. Maintain range of motion and biomechanical alignment.
3. Provide sensory feedback.
4. Increase the ability to regulate appropriate muscular force.
5. Decrease restraint to passive movement.
6. Improve the ability to reciprocate agonist and antagonist muscle contractions.
7. Develop a variety of movement and postural synergies.
8. Increase the adaptability of motor responses.

COGNITION-PERCEPTION

Physical rehabilitation of the stroke patient involves the relearning of a motor skill. The requirements for the motor relearning include (1) the ability to perceive the environment correctly, (2) the ability to focus attention, (3) the ability to understand instructions and the goal of movement, (4) an appropriate level of motivation, and (5) good memory functions of retention and recall.[26, 33]

The primary strategy to deal with cognitive deficits is to select the correct environment for motor relearning. The place of treatment should be quiet and nondistracting. Because many patients are easily fatigued and frustrated, frequent rest and periods of focused attention are the best ways to facilitate learning. Secondly, the patient must understand the goal of therapy. It is essential to have the patient's attention before giving commands. Instructions should be simple and supported by demonstrations and visual and tactile cues. Simple repetition and frequent cueing within the same treatment session and across treatment sessions are necessary for the patient with memory deficits.

Motivation may be facilitated by establishing goals that are meaningful and attainable. Patients must experience success in a treatment program and believe that what they have accomplished is important. Patient and therapist therefore should mutually agree on the goals for therapy. For example, the patient's goal for a treatment session may be to walk, and yet this patient may have not developed the necessary motor prerequisites. The therapist needs to explain her treatment strategy and demonstrate the relevance of the selected therapeutic activities to walking. Finally, the patient needs to be reminded to practice his new motor skills every day, so that he incorporates them into his ongoing functional activities.

Unilateral neglect of the hemiplegic side is a common problem in stroke rehabilitation. This neglect may be due to a perceptual deficit most frequently caused by a right-sided brain lesion, or it may be due to learned nonuse of the hemiplegic side. When hemineglect is present, it is important to continuously focus the patient's attention on the neglected side. Suggestions for management include (1) place objects on the patient's involved side, encouraging the patient to reach across the midline (Fig 6–1); (2) teach the patient to roll toward his good side, and encourage him to reach forward with his involved arm or leg (Fig 6–2, A) if he does not have sufficient motor function to accomplish this, let him assist his involved extremity with his less involved extremity (Fig 6–2, B); (3) in some patients, flashing lights or moving objects in the affected visual field may cue attention to the neglected side.

Perception of the environment is a critical factor for selecting motor strategies that can be used most efficiently to control posture and movement.[17] For example, if the patient's perception of vertical is abnormal, he will exhibit abnormal postural synergies and adaptation. A suggestion for intervention is to provide feedback (i.e., head position monitor, mirror with vertical line) to reorient the patient to the vertical.

Management of apraxia, or the inability to plan a motor task, is one of the most difficult aspects of stroke rehabilitation. Suggestions for intervention include (1) clearly explain the components of a simple motor task; (2) break down the motor task into basic steps, and have the patient practice (do it); (3) start with one step tasks and then gradually increase the number of

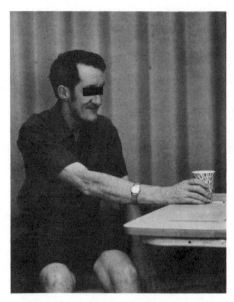

FIG 6–1.
Patient is encouraged to reach for an object on the affected side of the body. Attention and gaze need to be directed away from intact side in order to prevent unilateral neglect.

steps. Once the patient is able to perform several steps, ask the patient to independently organize and plan the motor task.

RANGE OF MOTION

Stretching and early mobilization of the stroke patient are the key to prevention of decreasing range of motion or contractures. Loss of mobility is minimized with positioning,[15] splinting,[22, 29] range of motion exercises,[27, 34] and active and functional use of the extremities. In stroke patients, rhythmic rotation, slow maintained stretch, or weight bearing in conjunction with active movement is effective in preventing future contractures.[31]

Current research has shown that biomechanical alignment influences the distribution, onset, and intensity of electrical activity in postural muscles.[3] In stroke, incorrect body alignment caused by decreased joint range of motion may be a primary source of abnormal postural adjustments and movement.

An example of a common range-of-motion problem in stroke patients is subtalar ligamentous tightness producing a rigidly supinated foot. A rigid mortis prevents weight shift over the forefoot in stance. A primary goal of physical therapy is to increase range of motion available in dorsiflexion and pronation to produce normal foot alignment and ankle motion. If the base is not in proper alignment, the rest of the lower extremity kinematic chain will be affected. With ankle range of motion and the feet placed in an appropriate position, weight shift and weight bearing on the involved extremity may be more likely.

Short leg inhibitive casting is a relatively new and frequently recommended technique for improving motor control in the lower extremity during stance and gait.[39] The scientific basis for using this technique is not clearly defined. We speculate, however, that this is a useful procedure, because it does provide more normal biomechanical alignment. This would directly increase the patient's ability to select a more appropriate movement strategy and produce more normal sequencing of muscle activation.

SENSATION

In stroke rehabilitation the therapist should assess which sensory systems are compromised and then select alternative stimuli to provide feedback about motor performance. All therapeutic techniques for stroke rehabilitation activate four sensory systems: visual, vestibular, auditory, and somatosen-

---

FIG 6–2.   →

A, patient practices rolling forward while reaching out with his arm. Therapist is guiding the movement. **B,** bilateral reaching is incorporated during rolling to assist scapula protraction and place the affected arm within the visual field.

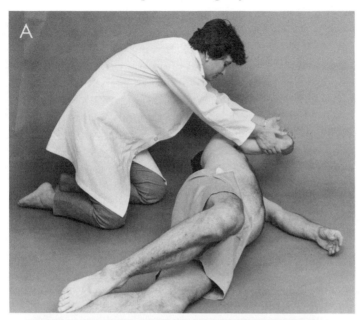

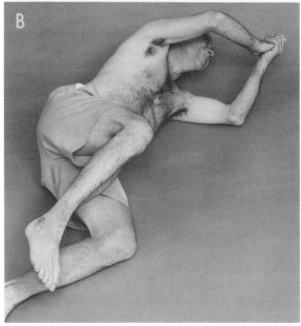

sory. If one sensory modality is impaired or distorted, the other modalities can substitute to provide feedback and facilitate motor relearning. For example, if the patient has decreased proprioception, visual and auditory cues can be used to increase the patient's knowledge of performance.[23] Touch, tapping, and quick stretch are a few examples of somatosensory cues that may reinforce a movement. Electromyographic biofeedback is an example of an external mode of sensory feedback that informs the patient about the consequences of his movement. This particular method has been shown to be particularly effective in stroke rehabilitation.[13, 14, 41] General guidelines for providing sensory information are (1) feedback should always be used in functional, goal-directed activities rather than in isolated muscle action; (2) sensory retraining should begin as soon as possible in order to minimize learned nonuse; (3) sensory training should incorporate much practice and repetition; and (4) feedback should be withdrawn when the patient has relearned a movement.[26, 33, 38]

STRENGTH

The patient must produce sufficient muscular strength to maintain posture and move. The strength produced by a muscle contraction may be optimized by providing the best biomechanical conditions for force production and using techniques that augment motor unit recruitment.

The biomechanical factors affecting muscular strength include type of muscle contraction, muscle length, velocity of muscle contraction, and moment arm.[35] In initial therapy, eccentric muscle contractions should be emphasized prior to concentric muscle contractions. Eccentric muscle contractions afford the greatest muscle strength with less demand for motor unit activity.[1] This subsequently increases the patient's chance for controlling the movement and decreasing the sense of effort. A second consideration is that the force produced by a muscle contraction is increased if the muscle has an optimal length/tension relation. For example, a stroke patient may be unable to generate any knee flexor torque when he is sitting with the hip at 90 degrees of flexion. However, flexor torque will increase and be functional if the patient leans forward, flexing his hip beyond 90 degrees. By flexing his hip, he increases the length of the hamstrings, which contributes to an increased force. Stroke patients have difficulty generating force at high velocities of movement. This is due in part to their inability to recruit fast-twitch motor units.[22] If the goal of therapeutic intervention is to increase muscle strength, then slow rather than fast velocities should be initially selected.

Finally, if the patient is unable to move through the range of motion, select the joint angle that affords the greatest musculotendinous moment arm ("perpendicular distance from the line of application of the musculotendinous unit to the axis of rotation of the joint"[35]). At this point in the range of motion, the patient may produce a functional force.

Many therapeutic techniques enhance motor unit recruitment, subsequently increasing the strength of muscle contraction. These techniques, which include tapping, vibration, stretch, resistance, electrical stimulation, and tactile stimulation, should be used in conjunction with voluntary effort.[7, 10, 11, 20, 21] Independent performance is the goal, and the patient should be weaned from the external stimuli as quickly as possible.

Finally, to increase muscle strength and endurance, one needs to consider a logical sequence of activities. This sequence includes the following: (1) use facilitory techniques as the extremities are passively moved; (2) ask the patient to attempt voluntary movement as assistance is provided; (3) once the patient has developed some volitional control during assistive exercise, ask him to perform unassisted eccentric exercises; (4) ask the patient to move against gravity; (5) withdraw all facilitory techniques; and (6) ask the patient to generate force against resistance repetitively and at different velocities. This strengthening sequence must not be continually performed in isolated movements, but rather incorporated into functional movement patterns.

MUSCLE TONE

The most important aspect of treatment of muscle tone disorders is to understand the specific pathophysiologic mechanisms behind the motor deficit. Key questions to answer are (1) is the restraint to movement caused by increased resistance to passive stretch (hyperactive stretch reflex), or (2) is the restraint to movement occurring during active reciprocating movements (abnormal regulation of the motoneuron pool for reciprocal movements)?

A great number of treatments are available to counteract abnormal tone in response to passive movement. Some of these are empirically based, but in others the mode of action has been scientifically established. Clinical modalities frequently used to reduce the resistance to passive movement include (1) cryotherapy, (2) slow elongation of the shortened muscle group, (3) weight bearing or moving the body on the affected extremity, (4) slow stroking, (5) rhythmic rotation, (6) inversion of the head, and (7) splinting or casting.[3, 12, 30] Again, we need to emphasize that these treatment techniques that reduce the hyperactivity of the stretch reflex may be beneficial in reducing restraint to passive movement, but may have little or no effect on active volitional movement. The temporary decrease in spasticity that occurs with any of these techniques does not directly effect an increase in function.[32, 40]

The restraint to active reciprocating movement is a more difficult problem to manage. This restraint is usually caused by prolonged recruitment of the motor neurons of certain muscles (i.e., flexors in the upper extremity and extensors in the lower extremity). Suggestions for intervention include the following: (1) facilitate contraction of the muscle antagonist to the overactive muscles; (2) do not reinforce contraction of an overactive muscle, because this causes prolonged recruitment and leads to an inability to reverse the direction of movement; and (3) practice reciprocation of movements in a slow, smooth manner.

Example.—A clinical example of minimizing restraint to active movement of the elbow is as follows: In the supine position, ask the patient to hold his forearm against gravity (isometric triceps contraction), lower the forearm slowly (eccentric triceps contraction) (Fig 6–3), and then lift the forearm against gravity (concentric triceps contraction). In this exercise, the patient has reinforced the triceps contraction without interference from the biceps. If the elbow had been actively flexed by the biceps, which are typically overactive, the patient would have been unable to reverse the direction of movement.

A third concept to consider when analyzing and treating abnormal tone is that during active movement, muscle activity increases dramatically when the patient has inadequate pos-

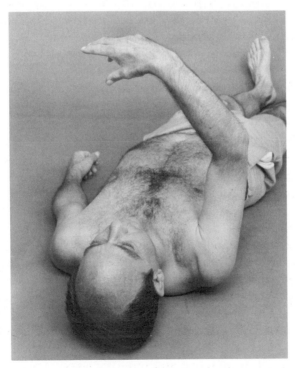

FIG 6–3.
Patient controls an eccentric contraction of his triceps in the midrange.

ture and movement synergies. For example, if the patient has abnormal postural responses of the lower extremity muscles, this will increase the effort necessary to maintain a standing position. In an attempt to prevent falling, the patient may recruit excessive and prolonged muscular activity to compensate for his postural instability. A goal of treatment may be to improve dynamic postural and movement synergies available, which would reduce the tendency for excessive prolonged muscle activity or cocontraction of muscles to stabilize posture.

In summary, the management of abnormal tone is an extremely complex process. The key to selecting appropriate intervention strategies is to more specifically identify the underlying causes of the "spastic" behaviors. The reduction of spasticity caused by hyperactive stretch reflexes is usually temporary and does not directly effect an increase in function. If during active performance, restraint to movement is caused by abnormal regulation of the motoneuron pool, then reducing the effort of the movement and encouraging smooth, reciprocal movements should carry over to functional movements.

SYNERGIES

The primary goal of treatment should be to break down the stereotypic movement patterns into smaller components of movement, then combine and reorganize these components to increase the patient's repertoire of movement options. These new patterns need to be finely tuned and expanded in order to increase their flexibility. This acquisition of selective control in hemiplegics requires five steps: (1) facilitate flexion and extension synergies; (2) mix components of the flexion and extension synergies; (3) develop and increase the number of postural and movement synergies available; (4) elicit the synergies volitionally as well as automatically; and (5) select appropriate functional activities and the most desirable environment in which to practice and reinforce synergies.

Movement is not an isolated process, but rather establishes a relation of the patient to the environment. A movement forms only one single component; it is just one element of an action. Therefore, it should be practiced in an action-related, functional context. The intention of the movement (action plan) is the determinant of the course of the voluntary movement sequence. An example of an appropriate sequence of activities for activating the hamstrings in a variety of synergistic movements might be as follows:

1. Knee to chest
2. Flex hip and knee during rolling
3. Prone knee flexion with hip extended
4. Sitting—knee flexion
5. Sit to stand
6. Propelling a stool forward with the involved extremity
7. Standing—hip extended, knee flexed
8. Pawing
9. Walking backwards
10. Gait

An appropriate movement strategy includes not only a plan of action for the ordered contraction of muscles, but also for the interpretation of the sensory feedback resulting from the performance (was the movement correct?). Synergies for attaining particular functional goals should be emphasized. Some patients are unable to elicit movements necessary in the context of functional activities. Such patients may need to volitionally contract the necessary muscles in the functional context, gradually reducing volitional control, and then learn to activate the response under different conditions (Table 6–2; Figs 6–4 through 6–22). We also need to determine if the patient is able to consistently select the appropriate synergy for the motor task.

In summary, the ultimate goal of treatment is to optimize the patient's ability to perform a variety of activities. Treatment strategies should facilitate the training of basic functional synergies.

TABLE 6–2.

Case Example: 38-Year-Old Man

1. *Observe*

   Patient does not shift weight over right foot and ankle as he attempts to stand (Fig 6–4). Functional implications are poor balance and abnormal gait.

2. *Assess*

   Cognition—Excellent, well-motivated patient without any perceptual deficits.

   Sensation—Within normal limits.

   Range of motion—Within normal limits.

   Tone—Normal in response to passive stretch and no significant increase in muscle activity as patient attempts weight bearing.

   Weakness—The patient does not have significant weakness. He can volitionally dorsiflex and evert his ankle in supine or sitting (Figs 6–5 and 6–6).

   Synergistic organization—The patient volitionally dorsiflexes and everts the foot with flexion and extension of hip and knee (Figs 6–7 and 6–8). However, this does not carry over in functional movement patterns (Fig 6–9).

   Adaptability—No automatic postural responses of lower extremity in sitting or standing (Figs 6–4 and 6–10).

3. *Evaluate*

   Primary deficit is the inability to elicit ankle musculature in the context of postural control and functional activities.

4. *Select Intervention Strategies*

   Considering the patient's young age, first stroke, good sensation, excellent motivation, and degree of motor involvement, a realistic goal for therapy is to normalize movement and functional abilities.

5. *Treat*

   Encourage the patient to volitionally contract the muscle in the context of functional activities (i.e., rolling [Fig 6–11], standing up [Fig 6–12], rolling a stool [Fig 6–13], moving away from a wall [Fig 6–14], postural disturbances [Fig 6–15], and volitional sway [Fig 6–16]. Gradually reduce the patient's cognitive attention to the task by decreasing the patient's voluntary initiation of the movement patterns. Then continue to reinforce with practice. Finally, increase the speed amplitude and adaptability of the response (Figs 6–17 through 6–19).

6. *Reevaluate*

   Assess patient's ability to use relearned movement strategies in functional activities of balance and gait (Figs 6–20 through 6–22).

ADAPTABILITY

In order to be functional, the selection and initiation of a postural or movement synergy does not depend only upon the immediate stimulus to move, but also upon past experience, current environmental factors, and future goals.[17] Therefore, we need to set up environments that challenge the patient in different aspects of his capacity. The therapist needs to change the environment and work under many different conditions in order to (1) help access and initiate strategies appropriate for the condition, (2) fine-tune, adapt and develop new strategies, and (3) help movements become generalized to other situations in order to improve function and flexibility. In addition to providing a variety of situations, adaptability of motor re-

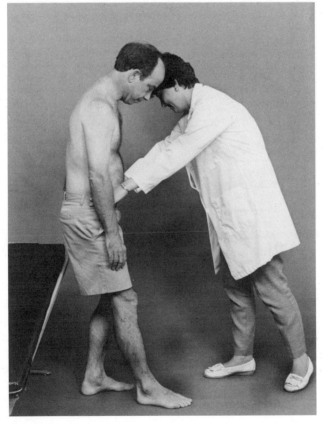

FIG 6–4.
Patient's weight is primarily on his uninvolved left side as he attempts to stand.

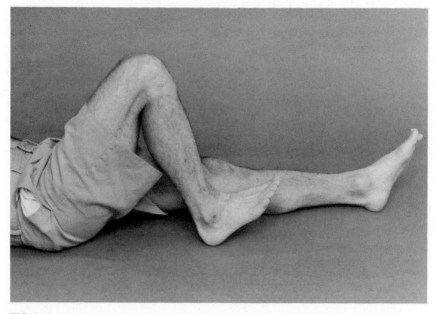

FIG 6–5.
Patient has been trained and is able to contract dorsiflexors and evertors in supine position.

sponses in stroke patients can be facilitated by requiring a variety of movement amplitudes, a variety of force requirements, and a variety of velocities.

Example.—A goal of treatment may be to increase the ability of the stroke patient to respond to subtle perturbations in the standing position. Once the response is correct, it should also be facilitated in other contexts (i.e., with and without vision, on foam and uneven surfaces). Velocity of the subtle displacements should also be varied. Finally, changing the base of support would demand new movement amplitude and force requirements.

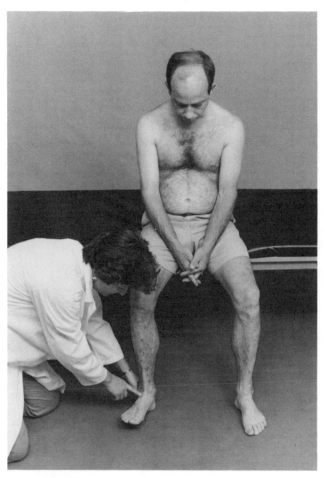

FIG 6–6.
Patient is also able to contract dorsiflexors and evertors in sitting position.

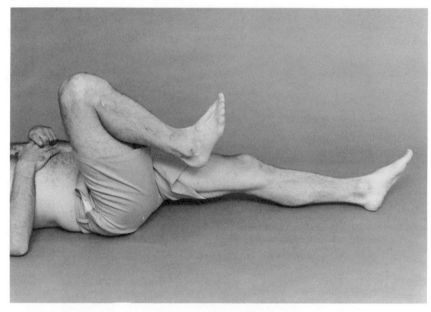

FIG 6–7.
Patient is able to selectively contract dorsiflexors and evertors with flexion of hip and knee.

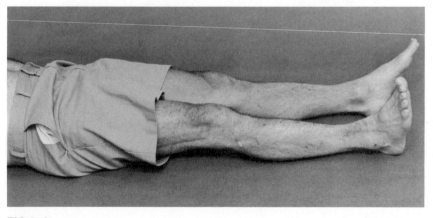

FIG 6–8.
Patient is also able to selectively contract ankle dorsiflexors and evertors with extension of hip and knee.

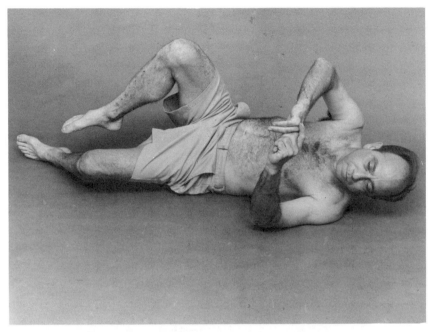

FIG 6–9.
Active ankle dorsiflexion and eversion do not automatically carry over in the functional movement pattern of rolling.

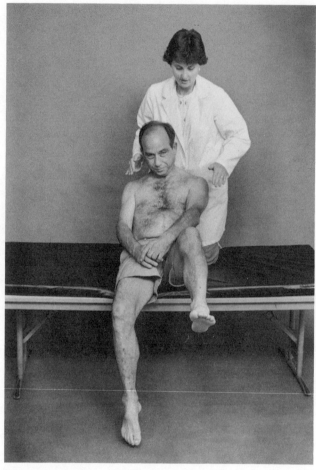

FIG 6–10.
Patient demonstrates no automatic postural responses of lower extremity
in sitting.

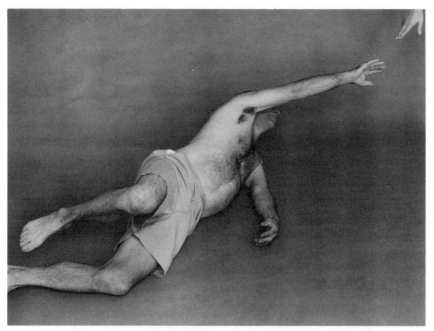

FIG 6–11.
Patient is encouraged to contract the ankle muscles in the context of rolling.

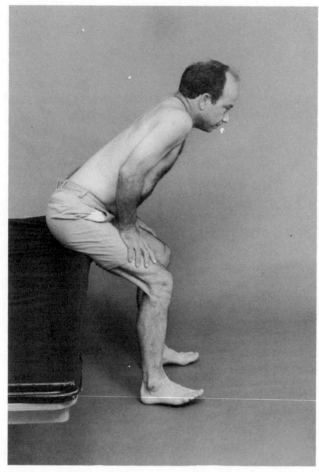

FIG 6–12.
Patient is encouraged to contract the ankle muscles in the context of standing up.

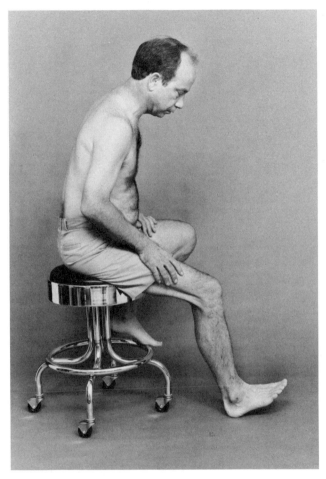

FIG 6–13.
Patient is encouraged to contract the ankle muscles in the context of rolling a stool.

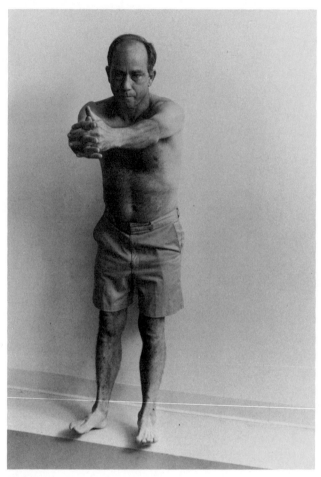

FIG 6–14.
Patient is enouraged to contract the ankle muscles in the context of moving away from a wall.

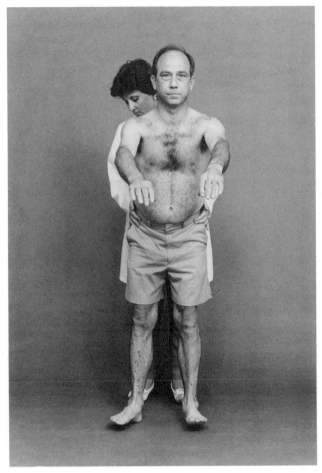

FIG 6–15.
Patient is encouraged to contract the ankle muscles in the context of postural displacements.

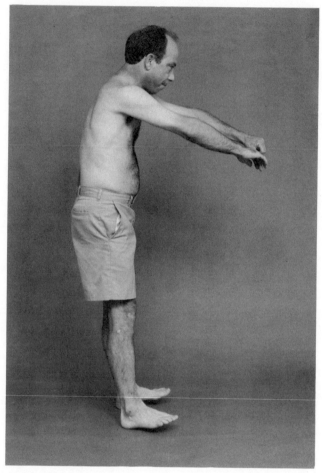

FIG 6–16.
Patient is encouraged to contract the ankle muscles in the context of volitional body sway.

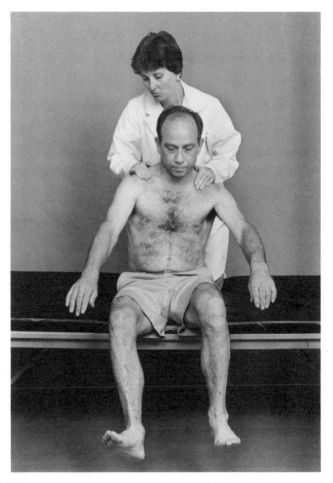

FIG 6–17.
Therapist asks patient to respond to increased velocities of postural disturbances in sitting.

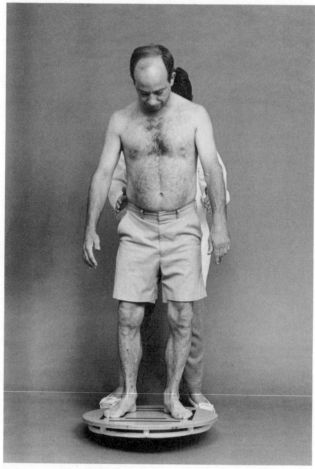

FIG 6–18.
Patient can increase speed amplitude and adaptability of responses on adjustable tilt board.

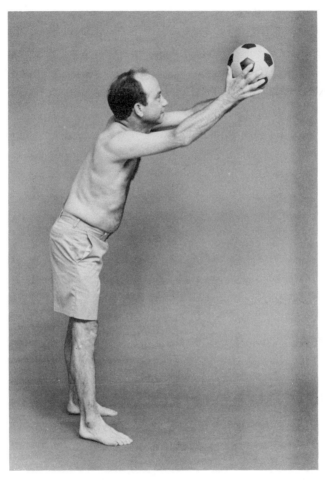

FIG 6–19.
Patient generalizes responses to other situations, i.e., throwing/catching ball.

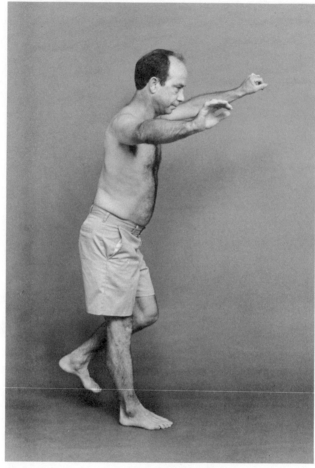

FIG 6–20.
Patient uses relearned movement strategies in balance activities.

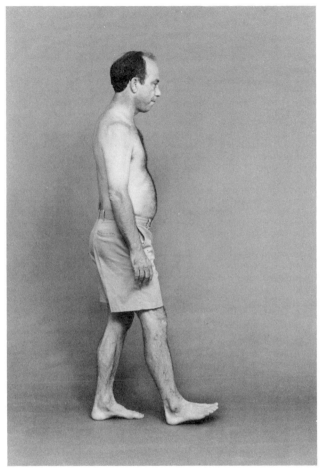

FIG 6–21.
Patient carries over movement during initial contact of gait.

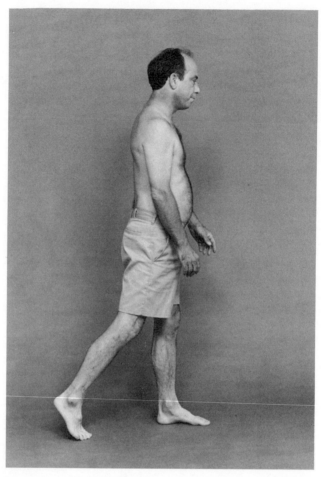

FIG 6–22.
Another example of patient using learned movement during preswing of gait.

SUMMARY

The successful rehabilitation of stroke patients depends on appropriate diagnosis of the movement disorder, establishment of realistic goals, selection of appropriate intervention strategies, and utilization of good principles of training and motor learning.

REFERENCES

1. Astrand P, Rodahl K: *Textbook of Work Physiology.* New York, McGraw-Hill Book Co, 1977.
2. Bach-y-Rita P (ed): Recovery of Function: Theoretical considerations for brain injury rehabilitation. Bern, Stuttgart, Vienna, Hans Huber Publishers, 1980.
3. Bach-y-Rita P: Brain plasticity as a basis for the development of rehabilitation procedures for hemiplegia. *Scand J Rehabil Med* 1981; 13:73–83.
4. Bach-y-Rita P: Sensory substitution in rehabilitation, in Illis J, Sedgwick M, Granville H (eds): *Rehabilitation of the Neurological Patient.* Oxford, Blackwell Press, 1982, pp 361–383.
5. Basmajian JV, Regenos EM, Baker MP: Rehabilitating stroke patients with biofeedback. *Geriatrics* 1977; 32:85–88.
6. Belenkiv Y, Gurfinkel VS, Paltsev YI: Elements of control of voluntary movements. *Biophysics* 1967; 12:135–141.
7. Benton LA, Baker LL, Bowman BR, et al: Functional electrical stimulation—a practical clinical guide. Downey, Calif, Rancho Los Amigos Rehabilitation Engineering Center, 1981.
8. Bernstein N: *Coordination and Regulation of Movements.* New York, Pergamon Press, 1967.
9. Binder SA, Moll CB, Wolf SL: Evaluation of electromyographic biofeedback as an adjunct to therapeutic exercise in treating the lower extremities of hemiplegic patients. *Phys Ther* 1981; 61:886–993.
10. Bishop B: Neurophysiology of motor responses evoked by vibrating stimulation. *Phys Ther* 1974; 54:1273–1282.
11. Bishop B: Possible application of vibration in treatment of motor dysfunction. *Phys Ther* 1975; 55:139–143.
12. Bobath B: *Adult Hemiplegia,* ed 2. London, Heinemann Medical, 1978.

13. Brudny J, Korein J, Levidow L, et al: Sensory feedback therapy as a modality of treatment in central nervous system disorders of voluntary movement. *Neurology* 1974; 24:825–832.
14. Brudny J, Korein J, Grynbaum BB, et al: Helping hemiparetics to help themselves: Sensory feedback therapy. *JAMA* 1979; 241:814–818.
15. Calliet R: *The Shoulder in Hemiplegia.* Philadelphia, FA Davis Co, 1980.
16. Carr, JH, Shepherd RB: *Motor Relearning Programme for Stroke.* Rockville, Aspen Systems Corporation, 1983.
17. Cordo, PJ, Nashner LM: Properties of postural adjustments associated with rapid arm movements. *J Neurophysiol* 1982; 47:287–302.
18. Evarts EV, Tanji J: Gating of motor cortex reflexes by prior instruction. *Brain Res* 1974; 71:479–494.
19. Feigenson JS, McCarthy ML, Meese PD, et al: Stroke rehabilitation: I. Factors predicting outcomes and length of stay—an overview. *NY State J Med* 1977; 77:1426–1430.
20. Griffin JW: Use of proprioceptive stimuli in therapeutic exercise. *Phys Ther* 1974; 54:1072–1079.
21. Harris FA: Facilitation techniques in therapeutic exercise, in Basmajian JV (ed): *Therapeutic Exercise,* ed 3. Baltimore, Williams & Wilkins Co, 1978.
22. Harro CC: Implications of motor unit characteristics to speed of movement in hemiplegia. *Neurol Rep* 1985; 9:55–60.
23. Herman R: Augmented sensory feedback in the control of limb management, in *Neural Organization and Its Relevance to Prosthetics. Symp Spec* 1973; 73-82041:197–212.
24. Inaba M, Edberg E, Montgomery J, et al: Effectiveness of functional training, active exercise and resistive exercise for patients with hemiplegia. *Phys Ther* 1973; 53:28–36.
25. Johnstone M: *Restoration of Motor Function in the Stroke Patient.* New York, Churchill Livingstone, 1978.
26. Martenvik RG: *Information Processing in Motor Skills.* New York, Holt, Rinehart and Winston, 1976.
27. Mossman P: *A Problem-Oriented Approach to Stroke Rehabilitation.* Springfield Ill, Charles C Thomas Publisher, 1976.
28. Mulder T, Hulstyn W: Sensory feedback therapy and theoretical knowledge of motor control and learning. *Am J Phys Med* 1984; 63:226–244.

29. Neuhaus BE, et al: A survey of rationales for and against hand splinting in hemiplegia. *Am J Occup Ther* 1981; 35:83–90.

30. Odeen I: Reduction of muscular hypertonus by long-term muscle stretch. *Scand J Rehabil Med* 1981; 13:93.

31. Ryerson SD: Hemiplegia resulting from vascular insult or disease, in Umphred DA (ed): *Neurological Rehabilitation.* St. Louis, CV Mosby Co, 1985, pp 474–514.

32. Sahrmann S, Norton BJ: The relationship of voluntary movement to spasticity in the upper motor neuron syndrome. *Ann Neurol* 1977; 2:460.

33. Salmoni AW, Schmidt RA, Walter CB: Knowledge of results and motor learning: A review and critical reappraisal. *Psychol Bull* 1984; 95:355–386.

34. Sharpless JW: Contractures: Pathophysiology, prevention and treatment, in Sharpless JW (ed): *A Problem-Oriented Approach to Stroke Rehabilitation.* Springfield, Ill, Charles C Thomas, Publisher, 1982, pp 62–66.

35. Smidt GL, Rogers MW: Factors contributing to the regulation and clinical assessment of muscular strength. *Phys Ther* 1982; 62:1283–1290.

36. Traub M, Rothwell J, Marsden C: Anticipatory postural reflexes in Parkinson's disease and other akinetic-rigid syndromes and in cerebellar ataxia. *Brain* 1980; 103:393–412.

37. Urbscheit N, et al: Effects of cooling on the ankle-jerk and H-response in hemiplegic patients. *Phys Ther* 1971; 51:993.

38. Wallace SA, Hagler R: Knowledge of performance and the learning of a closed motor skill. *Res Quart* 1979; 50:265–271.

39. Winstein CJ: *Short Leg Casting and Gait Training in Adult Hemiplegic Patients,* thesis. University of Southern California, Downey, Calif, 1984.

40. Wolf SL, et al: EMG biofeedback in stroke: a 1-year follow-up on the effect of patient characteristics. *Arch Phys Med Rehabil* 1980; 61:351.

41. Wolf SL: Electromyographic biofeedback applications to stroke patients. *Phys Ther* 1983; 63:1448–1459.

7

Measurement of Motor Performance and Functional Abilities Following Stroke

Pamela W. Duncan, M.A., P.T.
Mary Beth Badke, M.S., P.T.

FUGL-MEYER MEASUREMENT OF PHYSICAL PERFORMANCE

An objective and quantifiable assessment of motor function after stroke is necessary in order to identify motor problems, measure recovery of function, and measure effectiveness of treatment. A number of assessments have been used to measure sensorimotor recovery following stroke. Many of these assessments have involved muscle strength testing and clinical neurologic examinations. These methods have been criticized because they do not consider that the motor dysfunction in stroke is often dependent on limited synergies and the patient's position. Bobath[3] and Brunnstrom[4] developed assessment methods that qualitatively analyze motor recovery of stroke and take into consideration the influence of posture and loss of selective motor control. These assessment methods, however, lack numeric scoring that reflects the actual severity of movement dysfunction being measured. In addition, quan-

199

titative analysis of the results of these tests is not feasible, rendering them insufficient for research purposes.

Fugl-Meyer et al.[7] developed a quantitative assessment of motor function following stroke, which lends itself to statistical analysis for both research and clinical work. This assessment method, which uses the methods described by Brunnstrom, measures joint range of motion and pain, sensation, motor function, and balance. The assessment utilizes a cumulative numeric scoring system with the option of scoring some or all components. The maximum score for all components of the test is 226. The maximum motor score for the upper extremity is 66 and for the lower extremity is 34. The results of the assessment may be expressed as a percentage of the maximum score.

Validity and reliability of the Fugl-Meyer Assessment have been established. Fugl-Meyer et al.[7] demonstrated the validity of their assessment with 28 stroke patients by measuring recovery over time. Several researchers have demonstrated concurrent validity of this assessment. Fugl-Meyer found that the scores correlate well with activities of daily living.[8] This assessment also correlates with somatosensory-evoked potentials,[14] abnormal postural adjustments,[2] and temporal gait variables.[5] Duncan et al.[6] established intratest and intertest reliability for the Fugl-Meyer Assessment in a study of 19 stroke patients. Therefore, the Fugl-Meyer Assessment is a valid and reliable motor assessment that is useful in objectively measuring recovery of function and comparatively analyzing the effectiveness of therapeutic intervention.

The Fugl-Meyer measurements of the motor functions of the upper and lower extremity assess five stages of motor recovery. The five stages are described as follows: (1) reflexes recur; (2) volitional movements can be performed within the dynamic flexion and extension synergies; (3) components of the flexion and extension synergies can be mixed; (4) volitional movement can be performed with increasing variety; (5) the patient has maximum scores in stages 1 to 4. The assessment includes 50 different movements, and the performance is graded on a three-point ordinal scale: 0, the item cannot be performed; 1, the item can be partially performed; and 2, the item can be faultlessly performed. The complete test form and criteria for scoring are shown in Appendix A. Directions for administering the Fugl-Meyer are shown in Appendix B.

BARTHEL INDEX

The major purpose of stroke rehabilitation is to improve functional status. There is, therefore, a need to meaningfully define and measure the functional status of stroke patients. This information is important in assessing outcomes and making placement decisions. The method used to evaluate activities of daily living (ADL) should be objective, valid, reliable, and easy to use. Numerous ADL assessments have been used for stroke rehabilitation. One of these, the Barthel Index, appears to be the most widely accepted and researched.

The Barthel Index[15] was developed empirically by Dorothea Barthel and was used to measure improvement during inpatient rehabilitation. This index has been used in much stroke research and has been shown to be both valid and reliable.[1, 9–12, 16] Gresham et al.[13] compared the Barthel Index with two other ADL scales and concluded that the Barthel Index possessed certain advantages (sensitivity to change, easy statistical manipulation, and more clinical familiarity).

The Barthel Index and guidelines for scoring are presented in Appendix C and Appendix D.

REFERENCES

1. Alexander JR, Eldon A: Characteristics of elderly people admitted to hospital: Part III. Homes and sheltered housing. *Epidemiol Commun Health* 1979; 33:91–95.
2. Badke MB, Duncan PW: Patterns of motor responses during postural adjustments when standing in healthy subjects and hemiplegic patients. *Phys Ther* 1983; 63:13–20.
3. Bobath B: *Adult Hemiplegia: Evaluation and Treatment.* London, William Heinemann Medical Books, 1978.

4. Brunnstrom S: *Movement Therapy in Hemiplegia: A Neurophysiological Approach.* New York, Harper & Row, 1970.
5. Brandstater ME, de Bruin H, Goroland C, et al: Hemiplegic gait: Analysis of temporal variables. *Arch Phys Med Rehabil* 1983; 64:583–587.
6. Duncan PW, Propst M, Nelson SG: Reliability of the Fugl-Meyer Assessment of sensorimotor following cerebrovascular accident. *Phys Ther* 1983; 63:1606–1610.
7. Fugl-Meyer A, Jaasko L, Leyman I, et al: The post-stroke hemiplegic patient: A method of evaluation of physical performance. *Scand J Rehabil Med* 1975; 7:13–31.
8. Fugl-Meyer AR: The effect of rehabilitation in hemiplegia as reflected in the relation between motor recovery and ADL function, in *Proceedings of International Rehabilitation Association.* Mexico City, 1976, p 683.
9. Granger CV, Greer DS, Liset E, et al: Measurement of outcomes of care for stroke patients. *Stroke* 1975; 6:34–41.
10. Granger CV, Sherwood CC, Greer DS: Functional status measures in a comprehensive stroke care programme. *Arch Phys Med Rehabil* 1977; 58:555–560.
11. Granger CV, Albrecht GL, Hamilton BB: Outcome of comprehensive medical rehabilitation: Measurement by PULSES profile and the Barthel index. *Arch Phys Med Rehabil* 1979a; 60:145–154.
12. Granger CV, Dewis LS, Peter NC, et al: Stroke rehabilitation: Analysis of repeated Barthel Index measures. *Arch Phys Med Rehabil* 1979b; 60:14–17.
13. Gresham GE, Phillips TF, Labi MLC: ADL status in stroke: Relative merits of three standard indexes. *Arch Phys Med Rehabil* 1980; 61:355–358.
14. Kusoffsky A, Waddell I, Nilsson BY: The relationship between sensory impairment and motor recovery in patients with hemiplegia. *Scand J Rehabil Med* 1982; 14:27–32.
15. Mahoney FI, Barthel DW: Functional evaluation: The Barthel Index. *Md State Med J* 1965; 14:61–65.
16. Wylie CM, White BK: A measure of disability. *Arch Environ Health* 1964; 8:834–839.

APPENDIX A*

TABLE 7A–1.

Fugl-Meyer Measurement of Physical Performance

Name —————————————— History Number ——————————

Age ——————————— Address ——————————————————

Date of Cardiovascular Accident —————————— Phone ——————————————

Diagnosis ————————————————————————————

Aphasia ————————————————————————————

Sex ——————————————

Handedness ——————————

Significant Medical History ————————————————————————

Test Number —————————————— Tester ——————————————

*All material in Appendix A is adapted from Fugl-Meyer A, Jaasko L, Leyman I, et al: The post-stroke hemiplegic patient: A method of evaluation of physical performance. *Scand J Rehabil Med* 1975; 7:13–31. Used by permission.

TABLE 7A–2.
Fugl-Meyer Measurement of Physical Performance

AREA	TEST	Joint Pain/Motion		SCORING CRITERIA	MAXIMUM POSSIBLE SCORE	ATTAINED SCORE
		Motion	Pain			
Shoulder	Flexion	___	___	Motion Scoring	Motion 44	
	Abduction to 90°	___	___	0–Only a few degrees of motion		
	External rotation	___	___	1–Decreased passive range of motion		
	Internal rotation	___	___	2–Normal passive range of motion		
Elbow	Flexion	___	___			
	Extension	___	___	Pain Scoring	Pain 44	
Wrist	Flexion	___	___	0–Marked pain at end of range or		
	Extension	___	___	pain through range		
Fingers	Flexion	___	___	1–Some pain		
	Extension	___	___	2–No pain		
Forearm	Pronation	___	___			
	Supination	___	___			
Hip	Flexion	___	___			
	Abduction	___	___			
	External rotation	___	___			
	Internal rotation	___	___			
Knee	Flexion	___	___			
	Extension	___	___			
Ankle	Dorsiflexion	___	___			
	Plantar flexion	___	___			
Foot	Pronation	___	___			
	Supination	___	___			

TABLE 7A–3.
Fugl-Meyer Measurement of Physical Performance

AREA	TEST	SCORING CRITERIA	MAXIMUM POSSIBLE SCORE	ATTAINED SCORE
Upper and lower extremities	Sensation			
	I. Light touch	0–Anesthesia		
	a. Upper arm ____	1–Hyperesthesia/dysesthesia		
	b. Palm of hand ____	2–Normal		
	c. Thigh ____		8	
	d. Sole of foot ____			
	II. Proprioception	0–No sensation		
	a. Shoulder ____	1–Three quarters of answers are		
	b. Elbow ____	correct, but considerable		
	c. Wrist ____	difference in sensation compared		
	d. Thumb ____	with unaffected side		
	e. Hip ____	2–All answers are correct, little		
	f. Knee ____	or no difference		
	g. Ankle ____		16	
	h. Toe ____			

TABLE 7A–4.
Fugl-Meyer Measurement of Physical Performance

AREA	TEST	SCORING CRITERIA	MAXIMUM POSSIBLE SCORE	ATTAINED SCORE
MOTOR				
UPPER EXTREMITY (SITTING)	I. Reflexes			
	a. Biceps _____	0–No reflex activity can be elicited		
	b. Triceps _____	2–Reflex activity can be elicited	4	
	II. Flexor synergy	0–Cannot be performed at all		
	Elevation _____	1–Performed partly		
	Shoulder retraction _____	2–Performed faultlessly		
	Abduction _____ (at least 90°)		12	
	External rotation _____			
	Elbow flexion _____			
	Forearm supination _____			
	III. Extensor synergy	0–Cannot be performed at all		
	Shoulder adduction/internal rotation _____	1–Performed partly		
	Elbow extension _____	2–Performed faultlessly	6	
	Forearm pronation _____			
	IV. Movement combining synergies	0–No specific action performed		
	a. Hand to lumbar spine _____	1–Hand must pass anterior superior iliac spine		
		2–Action is performed faultlessly		
	b. Shoulder flexion to 90° elbow at 0°	0–Arm is immediately abducted, or elbow flexes at start of motion		
		1–Abduction or elbow flexion occurs in later phase of motion		
		2–Faultless motion		

c. Pronation/supination of forearm
with elbow at 90° and shoulder at
0° —————

   0–Correct position of shoulder and
      elbow cannot be attained, and/or
      pronation or supination cannot be
      performed at all

   1–Active pronation or supination can
      be performed even within a limited
      range of motion, and at the same
      time the shoulder and elbow are
      correctly positioned

   2–Complete pronation and supination
      with correct positions at elbow and
      shoulder

                        6

V. Movement out of synergy

a. Shoulder abduction to 90°, elbow
at 0°, and forearm pronated ————

   0–*Initial* elbow flexion occurs, or any
      deviation from pronated forearm
      occurs

   1–Motion can be performed partly, or,
      if during motion, elbow is flexed, or
      forearm cannot be kept in
      pronation

   2–Faultless motion

b. Shoulder flexion, 90–180°, elbow
at 0°, and forearm in mid
position ————

   0–Initial flexion of elbow or shoulder
      abduction occurs

   1–Elbow flexion or shoulder
      abduction occurs during shoulder
      flexion

   2–Faultless motion

(continued)

TABLE 7A–4. *Continued*

AREA	TEST	SCORING CRITERIA	MAXIMUM POSSIBLE SCORE	ATTAINED SCORE
	c. Pronation/supination of forearm elbow at 0° and shoulder between 30–90° of flexion _____	0–Supination and pronation cannot be performed at all, or elbow and shoulder positions cannot be attained 1–Elbow and shoulder properly positioned and pronation and supination performed in a limited range 2–Faultless motion		
	VI. Normal reflex activity	(This stage, which can render the score of 2, is included only if the patient has a score of 6 in stage V)	6	
	Biceps and/or finger flexors and triceps _____	0–At least 2 of the 3 phasic reflexes are markedly hyperactive 1–One reflex is markedly hyperactive, or at least 2 reflexes are lively 2–No more than one reflex is lively, and none are hyperactive	2	
WRIST	VII. a. Stability, elbow at 90°, shoulder at 0° _____	0–Patient cannot dorsiflex wrist to required 15° 1–Dorsiflexion is accomplished, but no resistance is taken 2–Position can be maintained with some (slight) resistance		

b. Flexion/extension, elbow at 90°, shoulder at 0° _____
- 0–Volitional movement does not occur
- 1–Patient cannot actively move the wrist joint throughout the total range of motion
- 2–Faultless, smooth movement

c. Stability, elbow at 0°, shoulder at 30° _____

Scoring is the same as for item a

d. Flexion/extension, elbow at 0°, shoulder at 30° _____

Scoring is the same as for item b

e. Circumduction _____
- 0–Cannot be performed
- 1–Jerky motion or incomplete circumduction
- 2–Complete motion with smoothness

10

HAND

VIII. a. Finger mass flexion _____
- 0–No flexion occurs
- 1–Some flexion, but not full motion
- 2–Complete active flexion (compared with unaffected hand)

b. Finger mass extension _____
- 0–No extension occurs
- 1–Patient can release an active mass flexion grasp
- 2–Full active extension

c. Grasp 1–Metacarpal-phalangeal joints extended and proximal interphalangeal & distal interphalangeal joints are flexed; grasp is tested against resistance
- 0–Required position cannot be acquired
- 1–Grasp is weak
- 2–Grasp can be maintained against relatively great resistance

(continued)

210 / *Pamela W. Duncan and Mary Beth Badke*

TABLE 7A–4. *Continued*

AREA	TEST	SCORING CRITERIA	MAXIMUM POSSIBLE SCORE	ATTAINED SCORE
	d. Grasp 2–Patient is instructed to adduct thumb, all other joints at 0 ° _____	0–Function cannot be performed 1–Scrap of paper interposed between the thumb and index finger can be kept in place, but not against a slight tug 2–Paper is held firmly against a tug		
	e. Grasp 3–Patient opposes thumb pad against the pad of index finger; a pencil is interposed _____	Scoring procedures are the same as for grasp 2		
	f. Grasp 4–The patient should grasp a cylinder-shaped object (small can), the volar surface of the 1st and 2nd finger against each other _____	Scoring procedures are the same as for grasps 2 and 3		
	g. Grasp 5–A spherical grasp; the patient grasps a tennis ball _____	Scoring procedures are the same as for grasps 2, 3, and 4	14	

IX. Coordination/Speed—Finger to nose
(five repetitions in rapid
succession)

a. Tremor _____

0–Marked tremor
1–Slight tremor
2–No tremor

b. Dysmetria _____

0–Pronounced or unsystematic
dysmetria
1–Slight or systematic dysmetria
2–No dysmetria

c. Speed _____

0–Activity is more than 6 seconds
longer than unaffected hand
1–2–5 seconds longer than unaffected
hand
2–Less than 2 seconds difference   6

**Total maximum score of upper
extremity**   **66**

TABLE 7A–5.
Fugl-Meyer Measurement of Physical Performance

AREA	TEST	SCORING CRITERIA	MAXIMUM POSSIBLE SCORE	ATTAINED SCORE
LOWER EXTREMITY (SUPINE)	I. Reflex activity—Tested in supine position Achilles ___ Patellar ___	0–No reflex activity 2–Reflex activity	4	
	II. A. Flexor synergy Hip flexion ___ Knee flexion ___ Ankle dorsiflexion ___	0–Cannot be performed 1–Partial motion 2–Full motion		
	B. Extensor synergy (motion is resisted) Hip extension ___ Adduction ___ Knee extension ___ Ankle plantar flexion ___	0–No motion 1–Weak motion 2–Almost full strength compared to normal	6	
SITTING (KNEES FREE OF CHAIR)	III. Movement combining synergies A. Knee flexion beyond 90° ___	0–No active motion 1–From slightly extended position, knee can be flexed, but not beyond 90° 2–Knee flexion beyond 90°	8	
	B. Ankle dorsiflexion ___	0–No active flexion 1–Incomplete active flexion 2–Normal dorsiflexion	4	

STANDING

IV. Movement out of synergy (hip at 0°)

   A. Knee flexion _____
- 0–Knee cannot flex without hip flexion
- 1–Knee begins flexion without hip flexion, but does not reach to 90°, or hip flexes during motion
- 2–Full motion as described

   B. Ankle dorsiflexion _____
- 0–No active motion
- 1–Partial motion
- 2–Full motion

4

SITTING

V. Normal reflexes

   Knee flexors _____
   Patellar _____
   Achilles _____
- 0–2 or the 3 are markedly hyperactive
- 1–1 reflex is hyperactive, or 2 reflexes are lively
- 2–No more than 1 reflex lively

2

SUPINE

VI. Coordination/speed–Heel to opposite knee (5 repetitions in rapid succession)

   A. Tremor _____
- 0–Marked tremor
- 1–Slight tremor
- 2–No tremor

   B. Dysmetria _____
- 0–Pronounced or unsystematic
- 1–Slight or systematic
- 2–No dysmetria

   C. Speed _____
- 0–6 seconds slower than unaffected side
- 1–2–5 seconds slower
- 2–Less than 2 seconds difference

6

Total maximum lower extremity score

34

TABLE 7A–6.
Fugl-Meyer Measurement of Physical Performance

AREA	TEST	SCORING CRITERIA	MAXIMUM POSSIBLE SCORE	ATTAINED SCORE
BALANCE	1. Sit without support ____	0–Cannot maintain sitting without support 1–Can sit unsupported less than 5 minutes 2–Can sit longer than 5 minutes		
	2. Parachute reaction, nonaffected side ____	0–Does not abduct shoulder or extend elbow 1–Impaired reaction 2–Normal reaction		
	3. Parachute reaction, affected side ____	Scoring is the same as for item 2		
	4. Supported standing ____	0–Cannot stand 1–Stands with maximum support of others 2–Stands with minimum support of one for 1 minute		
	5. Stand without support ____	0–Cannot stand without support 1–Stands less than 1 minute or sways 2–Stands with good balance more than 1 minute		
	6. Stand on unaffected side ____	0–Cannot be maintained longer than 1–2 seconds 1–Stands balanced 4–9 seconds 2–Stands balanced more than 10 seconds		
	7. Stand on affected side ____	0–Scoring is the same as #6		
		Maximum balance score	14	

TABLE 7A–7.
Fugl-Meyer Measurement of Physical Performance

Motor			Percentage of recovery
Upper arm _____	Maximum score _____		
Wrist and hand _____	Maximum score _____		
Total upper extremity score _____	Maximum score _____		
Total lower extremity score _____	Maximum score _____		
Total motor score _____	Total maximum score <u>100</u>		
Balance			
Total score _____	Maximum score _____ <u>14</u>		
Sensation			
Total score _____	Maximum score _____ <u>24</u>		
Joint range of motion			
Total score _____	Maximum score _____ <u>44</u>		
Pain			
Total score _____	Maximum score _____ <u>44</u>		
Total Fugl-Meyer score _____	**Total maximum score** <u>226</u>	**Percentage of recovery** _____	

APPENDIX B*

DIRECTIONS FOR ADMINISTERING THE FUGL-MEYER ASSESSMENT OF MOTOR FUNCTION

1. General rules
   A. Perform the assessment in a quiet area when the patient is maximally alert.
   B. The following equipment is needed: a low plinth or bed, chair, bedside table, reflex hammer, cotton ball, pencil, small piece of cardboard, small jar, tennis ball, stop watch, and blindfold.
   C. The complete assessment usually requires 20–30 minutes.
2. Joint motion and pain: Compare passive range of motion and joint pain to the unaffected extremities
3. Sensation
   A. Ask the patient if he feels the light touch of a cotton ball on both arms, the palmar surface of the hands, both legs, and the soles of the feet. Compare the qualitative sensation of touch with the unaffected extremity.
   B. With the patient blindfolded, examine the position sense of the affected joint. Test the patient's ability to recognize slight as well as large alterations in positions. The patient may respond verbally or by matching position with his unaffected extremity.
4. Motor function
   A. Give clear and concise instructions. Mime as well as verbal instructions are permissible.
   B. Instruct the patient to perform the required movement initially with the unaffected extremity.

---

*All material in Appendix B is adapted from Fugl-Meyer A, Jaasko L, Leyman I, et al: The post-stroke hemiplegic patient: A method of evaluation of physical performance. *Scand J Rehabil Med* 1975; 7:13–31. Used by permission.

    C.   Repeat each movement three times, and score the patient on the best performance.

    D.   Do not facilitate any movement during the testing; however, verbal encouragement is permissible.

    E.   Test the wrist and hand function independently of that of the arm. If necessary, the elbow may be supported in 90° of flexion during the hand tests.

    F.   Upper extremity flexor synergy: Instruct the seated patient to fully supinate his forearm, flex the elbow, and bring the forearm to the ear of the affected side. The shoulder should be abducted to at least 90°.

    G.   Upper extremity extensor synergy: Instruct the seated patient to adduct/internally rotate the shoulder, extend his arm towards the unaffected knee. The starting position should be that of full flexor synergy.

    H.   Lower extremity flexor synergy: Instruct the patient in supine position to flex his hip, knee, and ankle joint fully.

    I.   Lower extremity extensor synergy: For the position of full hip, knee, and ankle flexion, instruct the patient to extend and adduct his lower extremity against resistance.

5. Balance

    A.   When testing the parachute reaction, a firm push is given *unexpectedly*.

    B.   In order to score a 1 or 2 when testing balance on the nonaffected side, the patient must be able to lift the affected leg off the floor.

APPENDIX C

TABLE 7C–1.*

Barthel Index

		WITH HELP	INDEPENDENT
1.	Feeding (help = if food needs to be cut)	5	10
2.	Moving from wheelchair to bed and return (includes sitting up in bed)	5–10	15
3.	Personal toilet (wash face, comb hair, shave, clean teeth)	0	5
4.	Getting on and off toilet (handling clothes, wipe, flush)	5	10
5.	Bathing self	0	5
6.	Walking on level surface (or if unable to walk, propel wheelchair)	10 0*	15 5†
7.	Ascending and descending stairs	5	10
8.	Dressing (include tying shoes, fastening fasteners)	5	10
9.	Controlling bowels	5	10
10.	Controlling bladder	5	10

*Adapted from Mahoney FI, Barthel DW: Functional evaluation: The Barthel Index. *Md State Med J* 1965; 14:61–65.
†Score only if unable to walk.

APPENDIX D*

RATING GUIDELINES FOR BARTHEL INDEX

1. Feeding
    10 = Independent. The patient can feed himself a meal when someone puts the food within his reach. He must put on an assistive device if this is needed, cut up the food alone. He must accomplish this in a reasonable time.
    5 = Some help is necessary (with cutting up food, etc., as listed above).

2. Moving from wheelchair to bed and return
    15 = Independent in all phases of this activity. Patient can safely approach the bed in his wheelchair; lock brakes; lift footrests; move safely to bed; lie down; come to a sitting position on the wheelchair, if necessary, to transfer back into it safely; and return to the wheelchair.
    10 = Either some minimal help is needed in some step of this activity, or the patient needs to be reminded or supervised for safety of one or more parts of this activity.
    5 = Patient can come to a sitting position without the help of a second person, but needs to be lifted out of bed, or if he transfers with a great deal of help.

3. Doing personal toilet
    5 = Patient can wash hands and face, comb hair, clean teeth, and shave. He may use any kind of razor, but must put in blade or plug in razor without help as well as get it from drawer or cabinet. Female patients must put on own makeup.

4. Getting on and off toilet
    10 = patient is able to get on and off toilet, fasten and unfasten clothes, prevent soiling of clothes, and use toi-

---

*Adapted from Mahoney FI, Barthel DW: Functional evaluation: The Barthel Index. *Md State Med J* 1965; 14:61–65.

let paper without help. If it is necessary to use a bedpan instead of a toilet, he must be able to place it on a chair, empty it, and clean it.

5. Bathing self

    5 = Patient may use a bathtub, a shower, or take a complete sponge bath. He must be able to accomplish all the steps involved in whichever method employed without another person being present.

6. Walking on a level surface

    15 = Patient can walk at least 50 yards without help or supervision. He may wear braces or prostheses and use crutches, canes, or a walker, but not a rolling walker. He must be able to lock and unlock braces, if used; assume the standing position and sit down; get the necessary mechanical aids into position for use; and dispose of them when he sits. (Putting on and taking off braces is scored under dressing.)

    10 = Patient needs help or supervision in any of the above, but can walk at least 50 yards with a little help.

6a. Propelling a wheelchair

    5 = If a patient cannot ambulate, but can propel a wheelchair independently. He must be able to go around corners; turn around; maneuver the chair to a table, bed, toilet, etc. He must be able to push a chair at least 50 yards. Do not score this item if the patient gets score for walking.

7. Ascending and descending stairs

    10 = Patient is able to go up and down a flight of stairs safely without help or supervision. He may and should use handrails, canes, or crutches when needed. He must be able to carry canes or crutches as he ascends or descends stairs.

    5 = Patient needs help with or supervision of any one of the above items.

8. Dressing and undressing

    10 = Patient is able to put on, and remove, and fasten all clothing and tie shoe laces (unless it is necessary to

use adaptions for this). The activity includes putting on, removing, and fastening corset or braces when these are prescribed.

5 = Patient needs help in putting on and removing or fastening any clothing. He must do at least half the work himself. He must accomplish this in a reasonable time. Women need not be scored on use of a brassiere or girdle unless these are prescribed garments.

9. Continence of bowels

    10 = Patient is able to control his bowels and have no accidents. He can use a suppository or take an enema when necessary.

    5 = Patient needs help in using a suppository or taking an enema, or has occasional accidents.

10. Continence of bladder

    10 = Patient is able to control his bladder day and night. Patients who wear an external device and leg bag must put them on independently, clean and empty bag, and stay dry day and night.

    5 = Patient has occasional accidents, cannot wait for the bedpan or get to the toilet in time, or needs help with an external device.

8

Assessment and Treatment of Locomotor Deficits in Stroke

Jacqueline Montgomery, M.A., P.T.

Stroke victims remain a large client population for physical therapists despite the decrease in incidence of stroke over the last two decades. One can estimate from demographic studies that of all strokes that occur in the United States in any given year, at least 500,000 persons are disabled to the degree that they require rehabilitation services.[18]

A retrospective chart review of 123 consecutive stroke patients who received rehabilitation at Rancho Los Amigos Medical Center in Downey, California, during 1980 showed that 83% achieved either household or community ambulation.[13] This figure is representative for like groups of patients (moderately to severely involved) across the country[11, 20] and indicates the extent of the need for therapists with expertise in the assessment and management of hemiplegic gait dysfunction.

The purpose of this chapter is to describe hemiplegic gait abnormalities, their causes and consequences, and offer means for their resolution or diminution.

Customarily, gait is described in functional units (stance and swing periods) and by the actions or postures that occur within each unit and subunit. Historically, terms have been

223

used which describe these events as they occur in an individual displaying a normal gait. Generic terms have been developed by Perry and associates,[14] because they adapt to both normal and pathologic gait and are used in this chapter. For clarity of material related to hemiplegic gait, an explanation of this terminology is included as well as a brief review of selected aspects of normal gait.

TERMINOLOGY

The swing period is divided into three phases—initial swing, midswing, and terminal swing. Initial swing is that point when the limb is lifted from the ground to begin advancement for a step (Fig 8–1). Midswing follows until the tibia reaches a position perpendicular to the floor, which is when it has just passed the supporting limb (Fig 8–2). Terminal swing is that position when the knee extends to achieve step length and just prior to the foot making contact with the floor to begin stance (Fig 8–3). The functional phases of stance are initial contact, loading response, midstance, terminal stance, and preswing. Initial contact is a frozen moment in time that begins the weight-bearing period, depicting limb position when

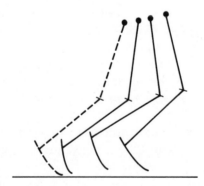

FIG 8–1.
Initial swing. The *solid line leg* represents the composite of this phase of swing.

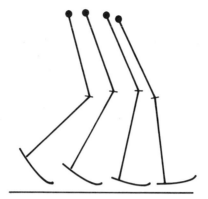

FIG 8–2.
Midswing.

the foot strikes the ground (Fig 8–4). It is quickly followed by loading response. Loading response is the reaction of the limb to the impact of weight acceptance (Fig 8–5). The next two stance phases—midstance and terminal stance—are the single-limb support periods. During midstance the body progresses over the foot while the opposite limb is advancing in swing (Fig 8–6). Midstance continues until terminal stance; when the body progresses ahead of the foot, weight is shifted onto the

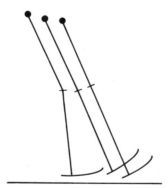

FIG 8–3.
Terminal swing.

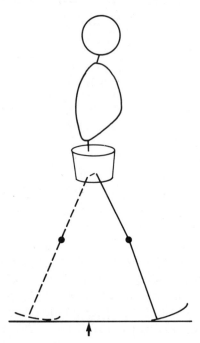

FIG 8–4.
Initial contact. The *solid line leg* represents the reference limb here as well as in Figs 8–5, 8–7, and 8–8.

metatarsal heads as the heel rises from the floor (Fig 8–7). During preswing, weight is rapidly shifted to the opposite limb just completing a step, and the stance limb is left in a trailing, toe-down position ready to repeat the cycle (Fig 8–8).

CHARACTERISTICS OF HEMIPLEGIC GAIT

A person disabled by stroke walks slower, using disproportionate step lengths with altered swing-stance time ratios and expends more energy for the same distance traveled when compared with a person walking normally.

Hemiplegics walk more than 50% slower than normal persons (37 m/minute vs. 82 m/minute),[24] have increased double-limb support time, which reflects decreased stance time on the

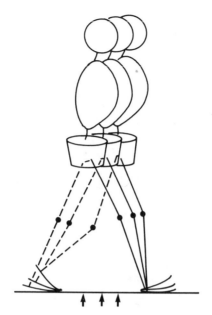

FIG 8–5.
Loading response.

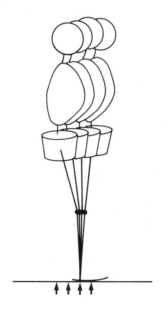

FIG 8–6.
Midstance.

227

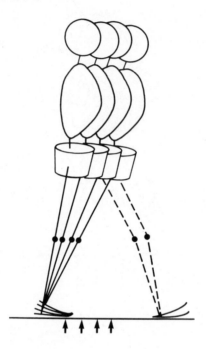

FIG 8–7.
Terminal stance.

more involved limb; and typically take a shorter step with the lesser involved leg. Although hemiplegics do not expend energy at a faster rate than normals, the energy demand overall is higher, because it takes longer to cover the same distance.[8, 24]

The characteristic electromyographic finding is the loss of normal phasic-modulated muscle activity. Although there are individual variations, three fairly distinct patterns have been identified. One is the tendency for flexor muscles to be active primarily during swing and the extensor muscles to be active primarily during stance in patients who clinically demonstrate pattern-only motor control.[2, 17] Another pattern is premature and continued activity of the stance muscles, and a third is a tendency for cocontraction patterns.[10]

Causes of gait dysfunction in the patient with hemiplegia are

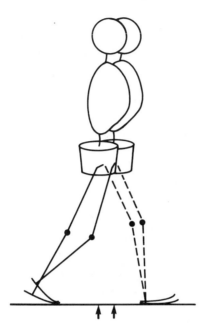

FIG 8–8.
Preswing.

impaired motor control and mechanical restraint such as soft tissue contracture. Loss of joint motion results from immobility and excessive muscle activity. Deficient motor control results from a myriad of neurologic sequelae associated with the site and severity of the CNS lesion. Abnormal patterns of limb motion often replace or predominate over normal selective control. Muscle activity may be reduced or excessive and prolonged. Deficits in postural reactions may include disorder in selection, amplitude, and timing. Integration of sensory information is distorted by impaired limb kinesthesia, deficient body image and spatial discrimination, and dulled tactile perception. Central balance systems may be impaired. Patients with a lesion of the posterior circulation may have truncal and limb ataxia. The interplay of these dysfunctions results in the loss of the preprogrammed control for automaticity in walking.

The consequences and significance of aberrant motor control will be illustrated by describing common hemiplegic deviations that occur during each gait phase.[16]

INITIAL CONTACT

The hemiplegic patient often lacks heel strike as the mode of floor contact, with resultant loss of the normal heel rocker action, which adds step length and assists in forward propulsion of the body. Instead, he lands first with his forefoot or with the sole of the entire foot. The causes are inadequate dorsiflexion to maintain the ankle at a right angle or incomplete knee extension or both. Usually, both causes must be present to result in forefoot-first contact.

Inadequate dorsiflexion may result from contracture, sustained and excessive plantar flexion muscle activity, the early activation of the triceps surae, which is characteristic of the pattern dominated patient, and inadequate dorsiflexion control (either selective or pattern). Both inadequate dorsiflexion and knee extension may result from pattern overlay, which prevents the combination of hip flexion, ankle dorsiflexion, and knee extension. Incomplete knee extension less frequently results from excessive hamstring muscle activity or incomplete range of motion.

Contact is made by the lateral border of the foot when the anterior tibialis remains overactive from swing or when the soleus is active as part of the premature activity of the triceps surae. The mode of floor contact influences the limb's reaction to weight acceptance in the subsequent functional unit of gait.

LOADING RESPONSE

There are two normal events during weight acceptance. One is rapid passive plantarflexion, which is restrained by the anterior tibialis and toe extensor muscles. This brief heel support period assists forward progression of the body. The second is knee flexion caused by the tibia moving forward faster than the thigh and serves to absorb shock from the impact of weighting the limb.

Varus and equinus are common problems in the stroke patient, with foot slap occurring less frequently. Foot slap can occur only if the patient has a heel strike followed by inadequate dorsiflexion control to resist the force of loading. This demand is considerably greater than the force required to lift the foot during swing.

Forefoot-first contact, caused by excessive plantar flexion, creates a significant problem during loading. Because the ankle cannot move into dorsiflexion, loading the forefoot forces the tibia back, creating a backward thrust into knee extension that impedes forward progression and the use of momentum to conserve energy.

Varus is caused by sustained activity of the anterior tibialis muscle (the only dorsiflexor involved in the flexion pattern[17]) or by premature action of the soleus. (The posterior tibialis is rarely overactive in a stroke patient.[17]) The result is an unstable, precarious surface for weight bearing. Relative varus occurs when overactive hip adductor muscles or imprecise foot placement from ataxia or deficient proprioception cause the foot to land in front of the opposite foot.

Knee reactions to loading depend on the initial position of both the knee and ankle joints and the type and amount of control of the quadriceps muscles. If the knee is in flexion at the beginning of loading and the patient has weak selective control and an available range of motion into dorsiflexion, the entire limb likely will collapse into flexion. If the patient's quadriceps reacts to weight bearing by reflex activation, sustained flexion without further collapse continues. If the patient lands with his knee extended (and often with his foot flat) and has inadequate quadriceps control (often accompanied by inadequate calf control), the knee will remain extended, because the patient will avoid all stance phase knee flexion since it represents a posture of instability (Fig 8–9). A knee extension thrust or hyperextension may be evident when forefoot contact is accompanied by high plantar flexion muscle activity.

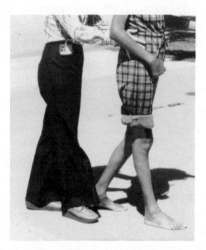

FIG 8–9.
Response to loading: knee remains extended with ankle plantar flexed as a result of inadequate quadriceps and soleus muscles control. (The patch above the patella is an electrode for muscle stimulation.) Note the abnormal terminal stance, preswing postures on the "uninvolved" side.

MIDSTANCE

Because midstance is a single-limb support event, the stance limb must support the full weight of the body while allowing mobility over a stationary foot. The primary demands are at the ankle and the hip.

During midstance the ankle moves from a position of 15° plantarflexion to approximately 10° dorsiflexion; the rate at which this motion occurs normally is controlled by eccentric contraction of the soleus. Controlled tibial advancement allows the knee to extend, following which the gastrocnemius then contracts to assist in restraining the tibia.

The knee extends to neutral in midstance by the ankle control described above, quadriceps activation in early midstance, and by momentum from the swinging limb.

Active hip extension continues from loading response, but quickly becomes a passive event as a result of the knee ex-

tending. Strong hip abduction activity occurs to maintain pelvic alignment as the opposite limb is unsupported.

Loss of ankle dorsiflexion mobility during midstance is a major source of gait dysfunction; causes are contracture, excessive muscle activity, and strong extension pattern. Two substitutions are used by patients who do not have adequate
dorsiflexion range (5°) to position their body weight over
their forefoot. Those with adequate range hyperextend their
knee. Others lean their trunk forward if they have adequate
hip extension control or if support is provided by a walking
aid. In both cases the pelvis is retracted and held back over
the heel or ankle, impeding both momentum and stride length.
It results in the characteristic shorter step of the lesser involved limb.

Another major problem at the ankle is inadequate soleus
muscle control, which results in uncontrolled tibial advancement. Patients with a strong quadriceps control will allow the
sustained knee flexion that accompanies the excessively flexed
ankle. Those with inadequate quadriceps control and sufficient
proprioception quickly learn to compensate by avoiding any
stance phase knee flexion, and the characteristic picture is persistent knee extension.

Common hip problems are inadequate hip extension control
to maintain the trunk in an erect posture and inadequate hip
abductor control to prevent a contralateral drop of the pelvis.
Patients with adequate proprioception and some selective control compensate by laterally leaning to the stance side—evident when they are not using an ambulatory aid that masks or
deletes the deviation. Most often they are unable to substitute
adequately.

TERMINAL STANCE

During the last part of the single limb support, body weight
moves ahead of the supporting foot with the heel off the
ground and the ankle in a neutral position from action of the
soleus and gastrocnemius muscles. Extension stability of the

hip and knee is by passive alignment; strong abductor activity continues to support the pelvis.

During terminal stance, there are three major functional deficiencies exhibited by the hemiplegic. The inability to advance body weight onto the forefoot results from contracture, excessive muscle activity or pattern, or pain from spastic, clawed toes. The characteristic deviation is lack of heel rise during single limb stance.

An excessively dorsiflexed ankle during terminal stance results from inadequate calf control. Body weight is not shifted until the opposite foot is on the floor.

The third deficiency, contralateral pelvic drop, results from inadequate hip abduction activity.

PRESWING

Floor contact by the opposite foot initiates this interval of double-limb support. The limb is rapidly unloaded, accompanied by passive knee flexion to 35–40° and approximately 20° of ankle plantarflexion. The toes remain on the ground as an assist for balance.

This subphase of stance is often missing in patients with inadequate stance stability, because they never get their limb in a trailing position. They often experience perpetuation of stance i.e., sustained knee extension rather than preparation for swing. Common deviations are limited or absent knee flexion because of the inability to advance weight forward and active knee extension as a result of excessive quadriceps activity or as a deliberate substitution for inadequate calf control (Fig 8–10).

INITIAL SWING

Normally, the knee actively adds 20° flexion to that attained passively in preswing, and the hip flexes 20° to begin limb advancement; both motions provide clearance for the foot and toes, which begin this phase in a plantarflexion position.

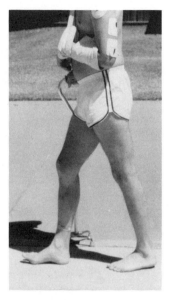

FIG 8–10.
Absent knee flexion and excessive dorsiflexion during preswing as a result of deliberate substitution for inadequate calf control.

The common hemiplegic problem is toe drag, most often caused by inadequate knee flexion, although it can be a combination of both hip and knee inadequacy. Patients attempt to compensate by circumducting their limb, or less often by vaulting on the stance foot or leaning their bodies backward or to the stance side.

Inadequate knee flexion is a result of insufficient preswing knee flexion, weak selective or flexion pattern control (the knee is usually the weakest component of the flexion pattern). Inadequate hip flexion is caused by inadequate hip flexor muscle action (selectively or in pattern) or because the dragging foot impedes it.

MIDSWING

Normally the limb continues advancement by unopposed hip flexor muscle action. Dorsiflexor muscle action raises the

236 / *Jacqueline Montgomery*

foot to neutral to achieve clearance as knee flexion passively decreases to 30°. At this point the tibia is vertical, and the foot is slightly ahead of the supporting limb.

The major problem for the stroke patient is inadequate dorsiflexion to clear the foot. Causes include plantarflexion contracture, excessive muscle activity, weak pattern, or selective control of the ankle dorsiflexors and toe extensor muscles.

Varus occurring only during swing is a cosmetic problem and may be caused by strong flexor synergy or inadequate toe extensor action to balance the inversion component of the anterior tibialis muscle.

TERMINAL SWING

The two changes from midswing that normally occur are continued forward rotation of the pelvis and active knee extension by the quadriceps muscles. Both motions contribute to step length. The hamstring muscles contract to restrain further hip flexion and counteract the action of the quadriceps to prevent knee hyperextension.

Patients who are dependent on stereotypic pattern control cannot maintain flexion of their hip and ankle while simultaneously extending their knee. Instead, they initiate extension to make contact with the ground and usually land in a semiflexed posture with the ankle plantarflexed. This action not only shortens their step, but puts them in a high muscle action demand posture to begin weight bearing. To increase step length or assist in reaching the ground, they may flex their opposite knee (with simultaneous dorsiflexion), creating dysfunction in the "uninvolved" side (Fig 8–11). A patient may lack full knee extension in terminal swing because of inadequate selective control of the quadriceps, hamstrings that are more active than the quadriceps control available, and excessive hamstring activity.

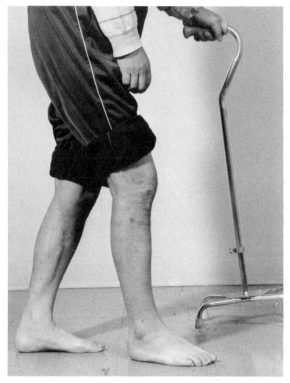

FIG 8–11.
Floor contact made with flexed knee and plantarflexed ankle in a patient who depends on pattern control. Note the short step of the right involved limb and the excessively flexed knee and ankle of the left "uninvolved" leg.

PELVIS AND TRUNK

Normally the pelvis moves through a few degrees of motion in three planes—forward rotation with the swinging limb during mid and terminal swing; slight downward drop just prior to initial contact; and posterior tilt at loading response, anterior tilt in terminal stance. These motions are passive, restrained by hip muscles. They serve to minimize the differences in leg length during a stride, reducing the body's displacement to 2 cm in each direction laterally.

Imperceptible motions of the trunk occur that minimize head displacement from the vertical; these motions, too, are passive.

These subtle motions are often lacking in the hemiplegic patient, giving him a stiff, robot-like appearance and contributing to abruptness of initial contact. The cause of these deficiencies is the loss of precisely timed eccentric contractions of the hip musculature.

EVALUATION OF GAIT

The single most useful tool in the clinical assessment of hemiplegic gait dysfunction is a skillful observer. Use of this tool presupposes a thorough knowledge of the postures, joint motions, muscle activity, temporal characteristics, and nuances of normal gait.

Prior to assessment and analysis of the patient walking, the clinician makes some preliminary observations. These include the patient's sitting posture and how he rises to standing to determine the extent of symmetric use of both sides of the trunk and limbs; standing posture and the degree of weight bearing on the more involved side; and the starting position and any changes with changed posture of the involved arm.

To critically analyze walking, the subject should be in clothing that allows viewing the alignment of the hips and exposure of at least the thigh distally; ideally the patient is barefoot. He should walk with as little support as possible to avoid masking deviations and creating artifacts.

One can systematically determine deviations by focusing first on stance deviations, phase by phase, joint by joint, and then proceeding in the same way through swing. Primary deviations are those that directly result from a deficiency such as inadequate segment control or increased muscle activity; compensatory deviations are those that result from deliberate substitutions made by the patient or as a secondary effect from a primary cause. An example of a compensatory deviation is when a patient circumducts his limb to substitute for inadequate limb flexion or when the knee thrusts into extension during loading as a result of excessive action of the plantar flexor muscles.

It is important to differentiate primary from compensatory deviation for understanding and analysis of the composite dysfunction and for planning treatment. One must understand the effect that change or correction of one segment has on another segment and determine if the benefit of the change outweighs the disadvantage. This is especially important in orthotic management and restriction of joint motion.

The clinician makes preliminary judgments about causes of detected deviations by constancy of their presence or when they occur during the gait cycle. For example, when ankle plantarflexion is present during mid and terminal swing and excessive dorsiflexion is present during midstance, contracture as a cause can be eliminated, and spasticity should be considered an unlikely cause.

Once preliminary judgments are made, one can proceed to selected standard clinical tests for verification or refutation. Because manual muscle testing is inappropriate for use in patients with upper motor neuron lesions, physical therapists at Rancho Los Amigos Medical Center have developed and use a test of limb control done in the upright position (Appendix). It was designed to test the patient in a position of function (standing); to incorporate the effects of upright posture and weight bearing; and to simulate activity required for walking, i.e., flexion that includes the factor of speed and extension, which assesses joint stability. Intertester reliability has been established at 96% agreement for flexion and 90% agreement for extension.

In 1983, Toman[22] completed a study designed to establish the validity of the Upright Control Test in predicting ambulatory function of patients with hemiplegia. Upright control scores of 20 patients with hemiplegia were compared with measurements of joint positions achieved, stride characteristics, and torque demands experienced during ambulation. Among his findings were (1) that test grades of weak and strong were more sensitive indicators of gait function than moderate grades—in fact moderate grades aligned closely with weak grades; (2) satisfactory relationships with gait achievement were ascertained in tests for hip and knee flexion, and hip and ankle extension; (3) strong hip flexion and extension scores appear to be key grades for functional ambulation; and (4) strong ankle extension control is a key contributor to velocity. As a result of Toman's findings, the factors of speed and repetition were added to the flexion test to more closely approximate the requirements for walking.

Other clinical tools used for overall assessment of gait include measurements of velocity, resting and immediately postwalking heart rate, walking efficiency, step and stride lengths, cadence (steps/minute), and endurance.

Results from these assessments are useful as baseline data to plan treatment, to measure progress, to help determine the most efficient means of mobility, and in some instances as prognostic factors.

Self-selected velocity (meters/minute) represents a cumulative quality score of a patient's ability and confidence in walking[6]; conversion to percentage of normal allows understanding by people of diverse backgrounds such as families and third-party payors.

Comparison of pre- and postwalking (at least 3 minutes) heart rate gives an indication of the demand placed on the cardiovascular system and the conditioning level of the patient (one must know if the patient is taking medication that alters heart rate). The relative cardiovascular efficiency of walking can be calculated and compared to a normal value.[19] Cardiovascular efficiency is determined by dividing velocity (meters/minute) by heart rate measured after at least 3 minutes of ambulation. Normal efficiency is 82%, based on normal velocity of 82 meters/minute divided by 100, which is normal average heart rate following walking.[24]

Endurance can be assessed by simple distance measurements coupled with time to determine practicality of walking as the primary means of locomotion. Lerner and Vargas[12] determined that it was necessary to cover at least 350 m in a metropolitan area to accomplish the everyday tasks of shopping, attending appointments for health care, and pursuit of leisure activities; they concluded that one must be able to walk that distance to be considered functional as a community ambulator. Patients who walk at velocities slower than 33% of normal usually do not achieve community ambulatory status, because it takes too long to cover the required distances.[1]

Step and stride length measurements can be made by a variety of foot and floor marking systems.[9] More sophisticated instrument systems are available.[21] One, the Veteran's Administration-Rancho Stride Analyzer, is a portable microprocessor-based computer system that can be used in a walking area at least 10 m long. It records foot-floor contact data obtained from foot switches, and calculates and prints out absolute and percent of normal values for velocity, cadence, stride length, single-limb and double-support time for each leg, and the percentage of time of the gait cycle for both swing and stance. The printout also records sequence of floor contact pattern for each foot.[15]

Dynamic electromyography, electrogoniometric systems, methods to measure ground reaction forces and torque demands at each lower extremity joint, as well as energy cost and photography systems,[21] are available in a number of gait laboratories across the country. Results are useful for assessment, treatment planning, and investigative studies.

MANAGEMENT OF ABNORMAL GAIT

Preambulation techniques are designed for the patient's mastery of four basic requirements or prerequisites for walking—upright balance (static and dynamic), the ability to alternately shift weight over the supporting limb, sufficient limb stability to support at least partial body weight, and the ability to successively advance each limb.

Emphasis of treatment is directed toward quality of control and movement—both in preambulation activities and gait training per se. Empirically, the highest quality of movement is achieved by use of techniques that foster normal postural reactions and patterns of movement; increase awareness and integration of activity in the trunk, pelvis, and involved extremities; demand weight-bearing and postural reactions on the more involved side; and promote early control over proximal rather than distal segments.

This approach to treatment is well described and illustrated by Bobath[4] and Carr and Shepherd.[7] The reader is referred to both sources for an in-depth explanation of this approach and specific treatment techniques. This system of treatment is augmented by additional methods that promote stability and improve the quality of movement—neuromuscular electrical stimulation[3] (NMES), orthoses, and selected resistance exercises. The criterion for their use is that their result is improved function through enhanced stability and movement. Selected problem areas and treatment suggestion examples follow.

Deficient static upright balance results from impaired body image or when a lesion of the posterior circulation causes a loss of balance backward with or without accompanying truncal and limb ataxia.

Deficiencies in body image are manifest as failure to shift one's center body weight over the area of support and failure to recognize nonsupport of an unstable involved stance extremity with resultant falling to the involved side. Significant deficiencies in both body image and backward balance problems are apparent during sitting, which is the appropriate position to begin treatment. Management of the former includes activities that encourage weight bearing on both hips and asymmetric weight bearing on the involved hip, such as sidesitting, leaning and reaching toward the involved side, and crossing the lesser involved leg over the involved leg. Reaching and leaning forward with the trunk and both arms (supported as needed) are appropriate activities for both problems, with progression to rising to partial standing encouraging bilateral weight bearing.

Initial upright activities begin with encouragement of equal double-limb support, which may need to be assisted by manual or appliance support for an unstable knee and manual assistance for appropriate head, trunk, and hip alignment. Treatment is progressed to lessening support, decreasing verbal and manual cueing, adding lateral weight shift, and then anterior and posterior stepping with the lesser involved leg while maintaining an erect trunk.

Once the patient has acquired the fundamental prerequisites to walking, forward progression is started with treatment directed toward major problems that interfere with stance stability.

TREATMENT TECHNIQUES FOR STANCE DEVIATIONS

INITIAL CONTACT

A patient can be provided with a heel-first mode of floor contact by several means, depending on the cause of the deviation. A simple drop foot resulting from inadequate dorsiflexors without moderate-to-severe excessive plantarflexion muscle activity can be corrected by an ankle-foot orthosis (AFO). The one of choice is made of lightweight polypropylene (1/8-inch thickness) at an angle perpendicular to the floor (when measured inside the patient's shoe to account for heel height) and enough flexibility to yield into plantarflexion for loading. This is preferred over a spring-assisted, double-bar upright type, because it is lighter (no shoe shank required), has more aesthetic appeal, and is interchangeable among shoes.

A method to facilitate adequate dorsiflexion for heel strike is the use of NMES triggered by a hand switch controlled by the therapist or by a footswitch placed in the patient's shoe sole.[3]

No heel strike as a result of excessive plantarflexion action with or without full knee extension is indicative of more overall limb involvement than a simple drop foot. Orthotic management of moderate-to-severe excessive plantarflexion muscle activity requires an AFO with a plantarflexion stop. Early postonset and extending into the months for neurologic recovery, the orthosis of choice is one with metal uprights and a double adjustable ankle joint. This is preferred over one made of rigid polypropylene, because its joints (i.e., ankle position) can be adjusted by the therapist. Requirements for this AFO are that it have an extended stirrup and be attached to a shoe with a shank that extends to the metatarsals (Fig 8–12). When one provides heel strike via an AFO, the patient's quadriceps control must be considered because of the knee flexion thrust that is created by the loss of plantarflexion. If the patient has marginal quadriceps control to accept this force, the heel of the shoe should be cushioned (Fig 8–13) or beveled (undercut). Even with stronger quadriceps control, this type heel provides a smoother transition into loading response.

When insufficient quadriceps activity contributes to lack of heel strike, their contraction can be augmented using NMES triggered during terminal swing. Cyclic NMES to the quadriceps inhibits excessive hamstring activity and is used to gain range of motion combined with stretching and positioning techniques or casting when a knee flexion contracture is present.

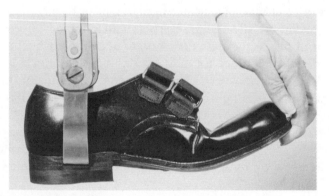

FIG 8–12.
The presence of a shoe shank that extends to the metatarsal heads (where the shoe bends with pressure applied) is required for an AFO with restricted ankle joint motion.

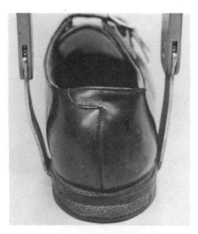

FIG 8–13.
Cushioned heel for a patient with a heel strike and marginal quadriceps control; it buffers the force into knee flexion by simulating plantarflexion. (From Montgomery J, et al: *Physical Therapy Management of Hemiplegia Secondary to Cerebrovascular Management.* Downey, Calif, Rancho Los Amigos Professional Staff Association, 1983. Used by permission.)

Correction of a varus posture in loading can be accomplished by several types of orthoses; selection of the proper type depends on concomitant problems. A flexible polypropylene AFO is effective as long as the lateral trim lines extend around the malleoli. Both a rigid polypropylene and a double-metal upright AFO correct medial-lateral subtalar instability unless they are fixed to the point that they are not correctable by manual force. In such an instance a lateral wedge and flare added to the shoe may be effective. Application to the shoe must include the point or location on the shoe where initial contact is made (Fig 8–14).

A medial orthosis made of flexible, moldable plastic can be used when mild-to-moderate varus is created by an overactive anterior tibialis. Use of NMES to activate the toe extensors and peroneus tertius, which balances the overactive anterior tibialis muscle, also is effective.

Other techniques to inhibit excessive plantarflexion activity include cyclical NMES to the dorsiflexors and evertors fol-

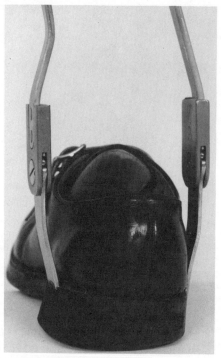

FIG 8–14.
Lateral heel wedge and flare when AFO alone cannot correct severe varus.
(From Montgomery J, et al: *Physical Therapy Management of Hemiplegia
Secondary to Cerebrovascular Management.* Downey, Calif, Rancho Los
Amigos Professional Staff Association, 1983. Used by permission.)

lowed by activities that include volitional control of those
muscles stimulated; foot mobilization techniques prior to
weight bearing; weight bearing with the ankle dorsiflexed; prolonged ice to the triceps surae followed by active exercise;
and serial or inhibitive casting. Serial casting has been shown
to be effective in both increasing range of motion and decreasing excessive muscle activity in patients following head injury.[5] Inhibitive casting is indicated for dynamic equinus or
equinovarus posturing. It incorporates the concepts of heel
and metatarsal weight bearing by use of a molded footplate

with recesses for the heel and metatarsal heads; prevention of abnormal posturing by fixed positioning in dorsiflexion and slight eversion; prevention of toe clawing by positioning in extension and abduction; and elimination of cutaneously reinforced abnormal reflexes. Although it has been used most extensively in children with cerebral palsy, several centers are studying its efficacy with adults.[29] Winstein's[28] study of ten hemiplegic patients showed those treated with an inhibitive cast had significant increases in velocity, single-limb stance time, and stride length over the noncasted subjects.

Fixed equinus with or without varus requires serial casting or operation for correction. Shoe adaptations that accommodate the deformity can be made when the patient is not a surgical candidate because of anesthetic risk or his choice. Surgical correction is considered during the period of neurologic recovery (no sooner than 6 months from onset) when the equinus or equinovarus is not correctable by conservative methods and after his clinical progress and neurologic status have plateaued. Equinus is corrected by lengthening the Achilles tendon; when varus is caused by an overactive anterior tibialis muscle, its tendon is split and transferred laterally to provide balanced dorsiflexion.[26] When the soleus is overactive, it contributes a varus force because of its insertion medially on the os calcis; its force is decreased as a result of the heel cord lengthening.

LOADING RESPONSE

Correction of foot slap depends upon increasing the strength and control of the ankle dorsiflexors to resist the force of loading. A flexible polypropylene AFO will control foot slap, but few patients will accept one when this is their only need.

The backward thrust of the tibia during loading caused by excessive plantarflexion action can be limited by a rigid AFO with a downstep as described under Initial Contact. Other techniques apply for loading response as well, including those described for excessive plantarflexion caused by increased muscle activity or contracture and those described for varus during initial contact.

Relative varus from overactive hip adductor muscles is approached by facilitation of hip abductors through static weight bearing in an abducted position, and using NMES if the patient has minimal adipose tissue to allow activation of the gluteus medius muscle. Serial anesthetic obturator nerve blocks using bupivacaine hydrochloride (Marcaine), which temporarily deactivates the majority of the adductor muscles, have proved to have some lasting effect as the patient gains increased abductor control. Relative varus from imprecise foot placement as a result of limb ataxia or impaired proprioception may be improved by weighting the extremity or using a training orthosis that prevents hip adduction via a joint between the pelvic band and thigh cuff.

When the knee goes into excessive flexion during loading as a result of inadequate quadriceps and soleus control, orthotic managment consists of a rigid AFO with a dorsiflexion stop.

Winchester et al.[27] determined by a study of 40 hemiparetic patients that positional feedback stimulation training (electrical stimulation combined with visual and auditory feedback) improved knee extensor torque for those patients receiving it compared with those receiving physical therapy without it.

Cyclic NMES to facilitate the major extensor groups (gluteus maximus, quadriceps, calf), as well as triggered, timed stimulation during gait, can be used. Other facilatory techniques for these muscle groups include sit-to-partial-stand, crouched-stand-to-erect-stand, "wall sitting," bicycling, and other resisted and reciprocal motions.

MIDSTANCE

Treatment of midstance problems begins with gaining proximal control during static double- and then single-limb support. If distal problems are present to the degree that a plantigrade foot is not possible or the ankle and knee are unstable, external support (AFO) should be provided. The patient is taught and manually assisted, if necessary, to proper alignment—trunk erect with normal lumbar lordosis, pelvis neutral, hip extended, and knee in neutral. The integration of this posture into gait facilitates extension control, and it is instrumental in gaining stance stability, allowing weight to be brought over the stationary foot; this alignment inhibits excessive activity distally, which results in equinovarus posturing and toe clawing.

As the patient gains proximal control for single-limb support, the joints of the AFO can be freed to encourage control of the ankle in an anterior/posterior direction when tibial instability results from inadequate calf control.

Although knee extension is usually the strongest component of extension, timing and duration of muscle activity is imprecise and not normally phasic in gait. Patients can improve timing and duration of activities by contracting through limited and varied arcs of motion.

As the patient gains static single-limb control, movement is added by stepping with the lesser involved leg to gain dynamic control needed for the single-limb support period of midstance. Manual upper-extremity support is provided and ankle control maintained by an AFO if required. Lateral hip instability from inadequate abductors, which results in loss of balance, can be helped by use of a cane.

Treatment techniques for ankle control problems are the same as described for initial contact and loading response.

TERMINAL STANCE

Toe clawing may be an additional problem in terminal stance that prevents body weight from progressing forward. A shoe insert that raises the metatarsal heads and spreads and extends the toes may alleviate the problem. Another means of correction is surgical release of the toe flexor muscles. If the long toe flexors are active throughout gait (determined by dynamic electromyography), they are released and transferred to the dorsum of the foot to augment dorsiflexion—often in conjunction with transfer of the anterior tibialis muscle.[26]

Adequate calf control is essential for simultaneous heel rise and weight forward over the foot, which are the characteristic features of terminal stance. Improved terminal stance can be achieved with an AFO, but it will not be normal because of the rigidity of the shoe and AFO that is required for ankle control.

PRESWING

This phase is often lacking entirely in a hemiplegic's gait. Its absence results from inadequate stability with inadequate lateral weight shift in the previous stance phases, which shortens the involved limb stance time; the inability to bring body weight forward because of control instability; excessive calf activity, which shortens the contralateral step; and inadequate trunk and hip alignment, compensating for instability of impaired sensation. Correction of these problems is required to allow the patient to have a trailing limb posture, which provides the alignment necessary for passive knee flexion and to begin initial swing from a position of advantage for activation of the hip flexors. Persistent quadriceps activity may interfere with passive knee flexion. If the rectus femoris or vastus intermedius show consistent nonphasic activity by dynamic electromyography during preswing and initial swing, one or both are surgically released to allow increased knee flexion.[23]

INITIAL SWING

Improved inadequate limb flexion is gained by improving stance stability, which results in a preswing phase and thus a trailing limb position.

Occasional benefits result from stimulation to the tensor fascia lata or to the peroneal nerve to activate a flexor withdrawal response. Weighting the extremity increases the arc of flexion when proprioception deficiency is the underlying cause. Reinforcement of flexion may result from resisted reciprocal or re-sisted bilateral motions such as proprioceptive neuromuscular facilitation techniques.

MIDSWING

Inadequate dorsiflexion for toe clearance can be corrected by any of the orthoses described under initial contact. The type of orthosis selected depends on other needs of the patient.

TERMINAL SWING

Side-lying, supine, and sitting activities that combine motions out of pattern are useful for the patient who demonstrates some selective control, but is dominated by patterns when upright. Progression to upright with resultant carryover into terminal swing is the goal. The use of triggered NMES to normally phasic muscle groups may facilitate the carryover process.

WALKING AIDS

Parallel bars are neither needed nor particularly useful during even the early phases of gait training for a patient post-stroke. Early standing activities are best accomplished from a mat, elevated as necessary (preferably one that has height adjustment), with the therapist in front of the patient. Parallel bars get in the way of needed mobility, and, if patients are allowed to use the handrails for support, they develop overuse habits of the lesser involved extremities.

Manual support from the therapist provides the best means of assisting and controlling the patient both in preambulation activities and early gait training. When an assistive device is introduced into treatment, one with wheels is preferred, because it allows continual forward progress without the start-stop influence of a cane or pick-up type walker. An adjustable-height bedside table with casters is useful for bilateral upper-extremity support (table top raised to elbow level) and encourages maintenance of an erect trunk. A progression from the rolling table is use of a supermarket-type shopping cart.

Many patients ultimately will need a walking aid to assist balance and provide support. Premature use, however, promotes lack of weight shift to the more involved side and development of stance stability. The aid selected for long-term functional use should provide the needed support and balance while allowing the fastest velocity with the highest walking efficiency value.

ORTHOTIC MANAGEMENT: INDICATIONS, TYPES, ADAPTATIONS, FIT, AND ALIGNMENT

The indications for several types of orthoses were discussed in the section on treatment for specific deviations; they are repeated here for emphasis.

The orthosis of choice for a patient with hemiplegia is an AFO, with the single exception of a patient who requires control of severe knee hyperextension. In this instance, a knee-ankle-foot orthosis (KAFO) (with a knee joint free to flex) is required to control the hyperextension. An external support that extends above the knee should be considered only as an early adjunct in gaining stance stability, and not for long-term orthotic management. If a patient fails to gain adequate knee and ankle stance stability enhanced by an AFO, he is not a functional ambulatory candidate. Further, use of a KAFO that locks the knee in extension requires that the patient compensate for denied-swing knee flexion, which adds to his disability; few patients with this degree of involvement have the bilateral arm and hand use and dexterity required for donning the orthosis.

Indications for an AFO include (1) inadequate dorsiflexion during midswing for toe clearance; (2) inadequate dorsiflexion for initial contact with the heel first; (3) medial lateral subtalar instability during any phase of stance (except varus at initial contact that quickly changes to plantigrade during loading); (4) tibial instability during stance; (5) uncontrolled foot placement as a result of impaired kinesthesia; and (6) postoperative protection for a patient who has undergone tendon transfer and postoperative positioning for a patient who has had a heel-cord lengthening.

Orthoses are indicated early postonset during gait training. Provision of distal (ankle and knee) stability during stance promotes proximal (pelvis and hip) control. Proper alignment during swing and stance facilitates appropriate temporal muscle activity. The selection of the type of AFO for any patient depends on the composite of his gait problems.

Correction of swing phase "drop foot" with little or no excess plantarflexion action can be accomplished by any of several available lightweight AFOs. The only one recommended is a posterior shell of polypropylene (1/8-inch thickness) made from a positive cast mold of the patient's leg.[25] The portion posterior to the malleoli in the area of the Achilles tendon is narrow to allow yielding for loading response. The major advantages of this AFO over others available are that it is durable and custom made for close contact with the foot and leg. It is lightweight, cosmetic, and interchangeable among shoes. Disadvantages include the critical nature of fit and the potential need for a wider shoe than the patient normally wears.

Varus during stance that is correctable manually also can be managed with a lightweight polypropylene AFO if the medial and lateral trim lines extend around the malleoli for support. This design, also custom-made, has the same advantages and disadvantages described above.

Patients with equinus or equinovarus posturing during swing and those with tibial instability require a more rigid AFO. An inflexible polypropylene (3/16-inch or 1/4-inch thickness) is suitable provided that the clinician knows precisely in what position the ankle should be fabricated (Fig 8–15). Once made, little adjustment is possible. It, too, is interchangeable among shoes, provided the original heel height is maintained. A larger shoe size is usually required. During early training it

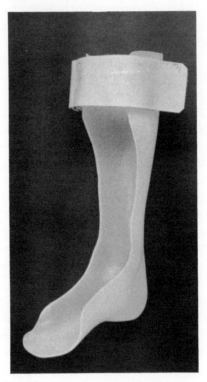

FIG 8–15.
Rigid polypropylene AFO. (From Montgomery J, et al: *Physical Therapy Management of Hemiplegia Secondary to Cerebrovascular Management.* Downey, Calif, Rancho Los Amigos Professional Staff Association, 1983. Used by permission.)

is prudent to select an AFO with adjustability to allow trial-and-error positioning and to permit changes as the patient's clinical needs change. The double-adjustable ankle joint AFO has metal uprights attached to the shoe via an extended stirrup riveted to a steel shank of metatarsal length in the shoe sole. A calf band of leather-covered metal secures it to the patient's leg at a height of about 1 inch below the fibular head. The design of this ankle joint allows considerable versatility. The therapist can make adjustments to provide free motion into both dorsiflexion and plantarflexion, to limit one or both, lock the joint at any position, or provide a spring assist into dorsiflexion. Therefore, depending on the needs of the patient, it can be adjusted to provide correction for any problem. Free motion is appropriate for a patient who requires control of varus only. A dorsiflexion spring assist is indicated for a patient who requires correction of only swing drop foot, although it is not the AFO of choice. A patient with equinus or equinovarus posturing during swing and/or tibial instability posteriorly during stance requires at least a plantarflexion stop. A patient with inadequate calf control and resultant tibia collapse during stance requires at least a dorsiflexion stop.

Patients requiring an AFO postoperatively need at least a plantarflexion stop. Polypropylene AFOs are not recommended postoperatively because of initial edema when the cast is removed and because of their lack of adjustability.

Another type of metal upright AFO is the single-adjustable ankle joint (Klenzak type); this has limited applicability. It is useful for the patient with primarily medial lateral instability (varus) without significantly increased plantarflexion muscle activity and commonly is fitted with a strong dorsiflexion spring assist with minimal limitation of plantarflexion. It is indicated for patients who, because of fluctuating lower leg volume or skin sensitivity problems, cannot use a closely fitting plastic AFO. The only adjustments possible by the therapist are removal of the spring assist and restriction of plantarflexion.

Various shoe adaptations provide support and correction that a shoe and AFO alone cannot provide. A lateral sole wedge plus a flare may be needed to correct severe varus. In order to be effective, it must be applied to the shoe at the point where the shoe initially contacts the floor. A lateral T-strap has limited use because of discomfort from the force required over the malleolus for correction.

A heel lift may be needed to accommodate an equinus deformity; it serves to angulate the tibia forward toward vertical.

Patients with spastic long toe flexors need a shoe with a high toe box to avoid skin irritation and breakdown over the dorsum of the toes. A custom-made insert that elevates the metatarsal heads and abducts the toes is useful in eliminating this posture.

For the infrequent stroke patient with valgus during stance, a molded medial arch support or molded plastic foot insert (University of California Berkeley Laboratory type) is useful.

The fit and alignment of any AFO are critical in attaining the desired effects. All types must fit comfortably, or the patient will not accept their use. Plastic AFOs should conform to the contour of the leg and foot without causing pressure, skin marks, redness, or irritation. The foot portion should extend just beyond the metatarsal head and support the foot medially and laterally. The vertical length of both plastic and metal varieties should be just distal to the fibular head. Metal uprights should be as close to the leg and malleoli as possible without causing pressure; the calf band should be closely contoured to the calf without causing restriction or pressure on the tibial

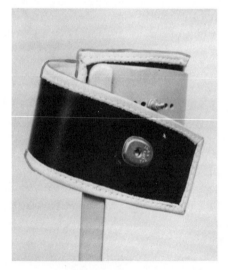

FIG 8–16.
Snap closure for the calf band of AFO. Note the adjustability provided by several holes for the button. (From Montgomery J, et al: *Physical Therapy Management of Hemiplegia Secondary to Cerebrovascular Management.* Downey, Calif, Rancho Los Amigos Professional Staff Association, 1983. Used by permission.)

crest anteriorly. The AFO should be attached to the shoe so that it is aligned with the anatomical axis of the ankle joint, i.e., with the medial joint slightly anterior to the lateral joint. This alignment is essential when there is motion provided in the ankle joint of the AFO.

Fastenings are important when the patient has limited dexterity or only one hand for application. Velcro closures or straps and buckles are acceptable substitutions for shoelaces when the patient can not master one-handed tying. A snap closure for the calf band can be managed with one hand and insures proper closure position, because it has been predetermined by the location of the button on the calf band. Several holes for the button are provided to allow for adjustment as necessary (Fig 8–16).

SUMMARY

The management of hemiplegic gait dysfunction begins with knowledge of the normal state for the basis of comparison. Analysis of deviations includes correlations with clinical findings for selection of appropriate techniques from state-of-the-art physical therapy and orthotic and surgical management to provide each patient with the safest, fastest, and most cosmetic and efficient means of locomotion available.

REFERENCES

1. Beekman C: Unpublished data.
2. Bennett P, Vandegrift C: *Study of Muscle Patterns in Hemiplegia,* thesis. University of Southern California, Downey, Calif, 1976.
3. Benton L, Baker L, Bowman B, et al: *Functional Electrical Stimulation—a Practical Guide.* Downey, Calif, Rancho Los Amigos Rehabilitation Engineering Center, 1980.
4. Bobath B, Bobath K: *Adult Hemiplegia Evaluation and Treatment,* London, William Heinemann Medical Books Limited, 1978.
5. Booth BJ, Doyle M, Montgomery J: Serial casting for the manage-

ment of spasticity in the head-injured adult. *Phys Ther* 1983; 63:1960–1966.

6. Brandstater ME, de Bruin H, Gowland C, et al: Hemiplegic gait: Analysis of temporal variables. *Arch Phys Med Rehabil* 1983; 64:583–587.

7. Carr JH, Shepherd RB: *A Motor Relearning Programme for Stroke.* Rockville, Md, Aspen Systems Corporation, 1983, pp 94–140.

8. Gersten JW, Orr W: External work of walking in hemiparetic patients. *Scand J Rehabil Med* 1971; 3:85–88.

9. Holden MK, Gill KM, Magliozzi MR, et al: Clinical gait assessment in the neurologically impaired. *Phys Ther* 1984: 64:35–40.

10. Knutsson E: Gait control in hemiparesis. *Scand J Rehabil Med* 1981; 13:101–108.

11. Lehmann JF, DeLateur BJ, Fowler RS, et al: Stroke: Does rehabilitation affect outcome? *Arch Phys Med Rehabil* 1975; 56:375–382.

12. Lerner MB, Vargas SD: *Determination of Functional Community Ambulation,* thesis. University of Southern California, Downey, Calif, 1983.

13. Montgomery J: Unpublished data.

14. *Normal and Pathological Gait Syllabus.* Downey, Calif, Professional Staff Association of Rancho Los Amigos Hospital, Inc, 1978, pp 2–11.

15. Perry J: Clinical gait analyzer. *Bull Prosthet Res* Fall 1974, p 188.

16. Perry J: Kinesiology of lower extremity bracing. *Clin Orthop* 1974; 102:18–31.

17. Perry J, Giovan P, Harris LJ, et al: The determinants of muscle action in the hemiparetic lower extremity. *Clin Orthop* 1978; 131:71–89.

18. Ryerson SJ: Hemiplegia resulting from vascular insult or disease, in Umphred DA (ed): *Neurological Rehabilitation.* St. Louis, CV Mosby Co, 1985, pp 474.

19. Schoneberger W: Personal communication.

20. Shafer SQ, Bruun B, Brown R, et al: Stroke: Early portents of functional recovery in black patients. *Arch Phys Med Rehabil* 1974; 55:264–268.

21. Smidt GL: Methods of studying gait. *Phys Ther* 1974; 54:13–17.

22. Toman CJ: *Upright Control as a Predictive Gait Measure in Pa-*

tients With Hemiplegia, thesis. University of Southern California, Downey, Calif, 1983.

23. Waters RL, Garland DE, Perry J, et al: Stiff-legged gait in hemiplegia: Surgical correction. *J Bone Joint Surg* 1979; 61-A:927–933.

24. Waters RL, Hislop HJ, Perry J, et al: Energetics: Application to the study and management of locomotor disabilities. *Orthop Clin North Am* 1978; 9:351–377.

25. Waters R, Montgomery J: Lower extremity management of hemiparesis. *Clin Orthop* 1974; 102:133–143.

26. Waters RL, Perry J, Garland D: Surgical correction of gait abnormalities following stroke. *Clin Orthop* 1978; 131:54–63.

27. Winchester P, Montgomery J, Bowman, et al: Effects of feedback stimulation training and cyclical electrical stimulation on knee extension in hemiparetic patients. *Phys Ther* 1983; 63:1096–1103.

28. Winstein CJ: *Short Leg Casting and Gait Training in Adult Hemiplegic Patients,* thesis. University of Southern California, Downey, Calif, 1984.

29. Zachazewski JE, Eberle ED, Jeffries M: Effect of tone-inhibiting casts and orthoses on gait: A case report. *Phys Ther* 1982; 62:453–455.

APPENDIX.—UPRIGHT CONTROL EVALUATION

UPRIGHT CONTROL (UC)

Criteria for performing UC evaluation (flexion and extension).
1. Patient requires no more than one person to assist double- or single-limb stance.
2. Patient can understand instructions adequately to perform test.

FLEXION

NUMBER OF EXAMINERS

Two examiners required for testing: assisting examiner provides hand support; testing examiner demonstrates test to patient and determines grade.

POSITION FOR TEST

Standing with use of assisting examiner's hand for support (balance only). Support should be sufficient for patient to maintain standing balance.

TECHNIQUE FOR ADMINISTERING FLEXION TEST FOR EACH SEGMENT

1. One demonstration by examiner.
2. One practice trial by patient (or two trials if needed to help patient understand test).
3. One test trial to determine grade.
4. If patient has bilateral lower-extremity involvement, provide opposite lower-extremity stabilization (manually, with ankle-foot orthosis [AFO], knee-ankle-foot orthosis [KAFO] as needed to provide standing stability.

PRETEST POSITIONING FOR HIP FLEXION TEST

Prior to the test for each segment:
1. Position the patient's limb that is to be tested in neutral or maximum available hip and knee extension.
2. The assisting examiner provides hand support in line with the greater trochanter of the femur on the side opposite the leg being tested.

INSTRUCTIONS TO PATIENT FOR HIP FLEXION TEST

1. "Stand as straight as you can."
2. "Bring your knee up toward your chest three times, as high and as fast as you can."

GRADING HIP FLEXION

(When observed range is borderline between weak and moderate, or moderate and strong, give the lesser grade. If patient is unable to complete the three flexion efforts within 10 seconds, give weak grade.)
1. Weak (W)—no motion or actively flexes less than 30°.
2. Moderate (M)—actively accomplishes an arc of hip flexion between 30–60°.
3. Strong (S)—actively accomplishes an arc of hip flexion more than 60°. (Base grade on true hip motion and not on substitutions such as backward trunk lean or pelvic tilt.)

INSTRUCTIONS TO PATIENT FOR KNEE FLEXION TEST

1. "Stand as straight as you can."
2. "Bring your knee up toward your chest three times, as high and as fast as you can."

Grading Knee Flexion

(When observed range is borderline between weak and moderate, or moderate and strong, give the lesser grade. If patient is unable to complete the three flexion efforts within 10 seconds, give weak grade.)
1. Weak (W)—no motion or knee flexes less than 30°.
2. Moderate (M)—knee flexes between 30–60°.
3. Strong (S)—knee flexes more than 60°.

Instructions to Patient for Ankle Flexion Test

1. "Stand as straight as you can."
2. "Bring your knee and your foot up toward your chest three times, as high and as fast as you can."

Grading Ankle Flexion

(When observed range is borderline between weak and strong, give the lesser grade. If patient is unable to complete the three flexion efforts within 10 seconds, give weak grade.)
1. Weak (W)—no motion or actively dorsiflexes to less than a right angle at the ankle joint.
2. Strong (S)—actively dorsiflexes to a right angle or greater at the ankle joint.

EXTENSION

Number of Examiners

Two examiners required for testing; testing examiner determines grade, assisting examiner assists in stabilizing or providing hand support as indicated under Pretest Position and Stabilization.

POSITION FOR TEST

Standing with the use of the examiner's hand for support (balance support adequate to maintain single-limb stance).

TECHNIQUE FOR ADMINISTERING TEST FOR EACH SEGMENT

1. One demonstration by examiner.
2. One practice trial by patient (or two trials if needed to help patient understand test).
3. One test trial to determine grade.
4. If patient has bilateral lower-extremity involvement, assist opposite lower-extremity flexion as needed to determine extension control of the stance limb.

PRETEST POSITIONING AND STABILIZATION FOR HIP EXTENSION TEST

1. Testing examiner positioned beside patient to provide hand support and to assure that patient begins from a position of neutral or maximum hip extension range.
2. Assisting examiner provides manual stabilization to maintain neutral knee extension and a stable ankle.
3. If there is a fixed equinus contracture greater than neutral, accommodate for the contracture by placing a 30° wedge under the patient's heel.
4. If unable to maintain a stable plantigrade platform for single-limb stance either manually or with an AFO, record UT (unable to test) for hip and knee extension. See Grading Ankle Extension for testing and recording an appropriate ankle grade.

INSTRUCTIONS TO PATIENT FOR HIP EXTENSION TEST

1. "Stand on both legs as straight as you can."
2. "Now stand as straight as you can on just your (R) (L) (weaker) leg—lift *this* leg up—keep standing as straight as you can."

GRADING HIP EXTENSION

(When patient is balanced on weaker leg, testing examiner gradually decreases amount of hand support to determine hip control.)

1. Weak (W)–uncontrolled trunk flexion on hip (testing examiner must prevent continued forward motion of the trunk by providing additional hand support).
2. Moderate (M)–unable to maintain trunk completely erect or at end of available hip extension range, but patient stops own forward trunk motion *or* trunk wobbles back and forth *or* patient hyperextends trunk on hips.
3. Strong (S)–maintains trunk erect on hip or at end of available hip extension range.

PRETEST POSITIONING AND STABILIZING FOR KNEE EXTENSION TEST

1. Assisting examiner positioned behind patient. Assisting examiner provides hand support and maintains trunk erect on hip.
2. Testing examiner positions patient's knees in 30° of flexion bilaterally.
3. If unable to maintain feet flat with approximately 30° knee flexion, use a 30° wedge.

Instructions to Patient for Knee Extension Test

1. "Stand on both feet with your knees bent" (approximately 20–30°; use a wedge to accommodate for limited ankle dorsiflexion range if necessary).
2. "Keep your knees bent and lift your (L) (R) (stronger) leg." Demonstrate and give instruction under number 3 *only* if patient can support body weight on a flexed knee during single-limb support without further collapse into flexion.
3. "Now straighten your knee as much as you can."

Grading Knee Extension Control

(If knee flexion contracture is present, grade cannot exceed "moderate.")
1. Weak (W)–unable to maintain body weight on a flexed knee (knee continues to collapse into flexion or heel rises).
2. Moderate (M)–supports body weight on a flexed knee without further collapse into flexion or without heel rise.
3. Strong (S)–supports body weight on a flexed knee and upon request straightens knee to end of available knee extension range (hyperextension allowed).
4. Excessive (E)–unable to position knee in flexion secondary to severe extensor thrust or extensor tone.

Pretest Positioning and Stabilization for Ankle Extension Test

If patient has knee flexion contracture, record UT (unable to test) for ankle extension control.
1. Assisting examiner positioned behind patient to maintain trunk erect on hip.
2. Testing examiner positioned to prevent knee hyperextension, i.e., plantarflexion of ankle.

3. Assess passive ankle range with knee extended and accommodate for neutral or less-than-neutral ankle range with a 30° wedge.

Instructions to Patient for Ankle Extension Test

1. "Stand on both legs as straight as you can."
2. "Lift and hold up your (L) (R) (stronger leg)." Demonstrate and give instructions for number 3 *only* if patient can control the knee at neutral.
3. "Keep your knee straight and go up on your toes as high as you can."

Grading Ankle Extension

1. Weak (W)—unable to maintain knee at neutral (knee collapses into flexion or wobbles back and forth between flexion and extension *or* hypertension/extensor thrust cannot be controlled by examiner).
2. Strong (S)—maintains knee at neutral and lifts heel off floor on command (any degree of heel lift while maintaining neutral knee).
3. Excessive (E)—equinus or varus so severe that patient is unable to maintain stable plantigrade platform.

Index

267